Perspectives
in Behavioral Medicine
THE AGING DIMENSION

Perspectives in Behavioral Medicine

THE AGING DIMENSION

Edited by

Matilda White Riley
National Institute on Aging

Joseph D. Matarazzo
Oregon Health Sciences University

Andrew Baum
Uniformed Services University of the Health Sciences

LEA LAWRENCE ERLBAUM ASSOCIATES, PUBLISHERS
1987   Hillsdale, New Jersey   London

Lawrence Erlbaum Associates, Inc., Publishers
365 Broadway
Hillsdale, New Jersey 07642

Library of Congress Cataloging-in-Publication Data

The Aging dimension.

(Perspectives in behavioral medicine)
Based on a conference held by June 5–8, 1983 in Reston, VA.
and co-sponsored by the National Institute on Aging.
Includings bibliographies and index.
1. Aging—Physiological aspects. I. Riley, Matilda
White, 1911–   . II. Matarazzo, Joseph D. III. Baum,
Andrew. IV. National Institute on Aging.   V. Series:
Perspectives on behavioral medicine. [DNLM: 1. Aging—
congresses. 2. Behavior—congresses. WT 104 A26745 1983]
QP86.A3594 1987   612'.67   87-8873
ISBN 0-89859-927-X

Printed in the United States of America
10 9 8 7 6 5 4 3 2 1

CONTENTS

LIST OF CONTRIBUTORS

DAVID ARENBERG   S-110 National Institute of Health, 4940 Eastern Avenue, Baltimore, MD 21224

ANDREW BAUM   Department of Medical Psychology, USU School of Medicine, 4301 Jones Bridge Road, Bethesda, MD 20814-4799

NORMAN S. BRAVEMAN   National Heart, Lung and Blood Institute, Westwood Building, 5333 Westbard Avenue, Bethesda, MD 20205

CHERYL CASHMAN   Department of Psychology, Yale University, New Haven, CT 06520

LAURIE DESIDERATO   Department of Psychology, Yale University, New Haven, CT 06520

CALEB E. FINCH   University of Southern California, Andrus Gerontology Center, Department of Biological Sciences, Los Angeles, CA 94305

STEVEN E. KELLER   Department of Psychiatry, Mount Sinai School of Medicine of the City University of New York, One Gustave L. Levy Place, New York, NY 10029

GEORGE L. MADDOX   University Council on Aging and Human Development, Duke University, Box 2920, Durham, NC 27710

JOSEPH D. MATARAZZO   Department of Medical Psychology, School of Medicine, Oregon Health Sciences University, Portland, OR 97201

JUDITH RODIN   Department of Psychology, Yale University, New Haven, CT 06520

MATILDA WHITE RILEY   Associate Director, National Institute on Aging, National Institute on Aging, National Institute of Health, 9000 Rockville Pike, Building 31, Bethesda, MD 20205

K. WARNER SCHAIE   S-110 Human Development Building, Pennsylvania State University, University Park, PA 16802

STEVEN J. SCHLEIFER   Department of Psychiatry, The Mount Sinai School of Medicine of the City University of New York, One Gustave L. Levy Place, New York, NY 10029

EDWARD L. SCHNEIDER   Associate Director for Biochemical and Clinical Medicine, National Institute on Aging, National Institute of Health, 9000 Rockville Pike, Building 32, Bethesda, MD 20205

MARVIN STEIN   Professor and Chairman, Department of Psychiatry, The Mount Sinai School of Medicine of the City University of New York, One Gustave L. Levy Place, New York, NY 10029

RICHARD F. THOMPSON   Department of Psychology, Stanford University, Jordon Hall, Building 420, Stanford, CA 94305

DIANA S. WOODRUFF-PAK   Department of Psychology, Temple University, Philadelphia, PA 19122

PREFACE

This volume, and the working conference that preceded it, break new ground in addressing the complex topic of aging, health, and behavior. Taking a bio-behavioral approach to a range of topics, contributors to this book have advanced their disciplines. The goals of the series *Perspectives in Behavioral Medicine* are generally to press forward in searching for important interfaces between behavior and health. In the present volume this general goal has been supplemented by addition of the dynamic aspect of aging. Cells, organ systems, and whole human beings all change as they move through life, linking health in varied and intricate ways to changes in behavior patterns, social structures, and cultural values and norms.

One characteristic of aging helps to make it important and exciting to study but also makes studying it more challenging and difficult. Aging is a classic biobehavioral construct. Few topics of study demonstrate the continuous inter-twining of biological and psychological processes that are revealed in growth and maturation of an organism. This is evident at all stages of life, but seems less evident in adulthood, perhaps due to the impressive array of conditioned responses and repertoires that adults carry around with them. However, as the writers in this volume suggest, the two are necessarily related.

This association suggests that the study of aging and health should be inter-disciplinary, and the approach taken in this volume is consistent with this. Scientists from a number of biological and behavioral science disciplines are represented. The working conference that served as the initiating event for this volume was made more exciting by the diversity of orientations and views that were present. The conference, cosponsored by the National Institute on Aging, was held in Reston, Virginia, June 5–8, 1983. Its purpose was to stimulate new approaches to the crucial, distant goal of understanding how aging processes, both biological and psychosocial, affect health. Harbingers of such approaches were the references to aging in the earlier reports by the Surgeon General on *Healthy People* and the Institute of Medicine on *Health and Behavior*. The conference format juxtaposed biomedical with psychosocial speakers, who brought their special expertise to bear on selected aspects of aging. Each set of formal papers was followed by workshop discussions aimed to involve members from various disciplines to define themes of common interdisciplinary relevance and topics ripe for interdisciplinary research endeavors. Benefiting from this interchange, most of the papers were rewritten after the meeting and reflect subsequent interpretation as well as the content that was presented.

The volume contains chapters that are based on presentations and discussion at the conference as well as chapters that were solicited after the meeting to balance or fill holes identified there. The resulting collection of papers will be of interest to students, researchers, professionals, and policymakers concerned with the aging process, the status of older people in society, or behavioral medicine in any of its forms. Health psychology, medical sociology, neuroscience, clinical medicine, and other disciplines or subdisciplines will all find much of relevance here. The chapters are uneven in the depth and extent of coverage of various topics. Some are broad overviews, others are briefer notes, exhortations, or presentation of findings. Some are detailed reviews, others are more speculative or data-based discussions. Yet the very unevenness of the chapters reflect the state of the art. It demonstrates the difficulty, but also the feasibility, of communicating from one discipline to another. It underscores the pressing need for defining and pursuing relevant research objectives at the nexus of health behaviors and aging. The time is ripe. The challenge is before us. Hopefully, readers will find material in this volume valuable for taking the next steps.

ACKNOWLEDGMENTS

Thanks go to the authors of the papers, most especially to those who are not themselves members of the Academy. Noteworthy are contributions from Norman Bravemen and Warner Schaie, who filled important gaps in the book by preparing papers after the conference was over. The editors appreciate the support of the other members of the Program Committee: Alan Herd, Jerome E. Singer, Ronald Abeles, Robert Ader, and John Riley. We are also grateful to Martha Gisriel for her tireless efforts on behalf of this book.

Perspectives
in Behavioral Medicine
THE AGING DIMENSION

1

AGING, HEALTH, AND SOCIAL CHANGE

An Overview

Matilda White Riley
National Institute on Aging

Our purpose in this volume, as in the working conference which it reports, is not merely to continue what the Academy of Behavioral Medicine Research has done so well—to develop the cutting edge of our dual perspective on biomedical and psychosocial research. Rather our hope is to take a further leap ahead. To remind us of where we began, I quote the statement of behavioral medicine from Neal Miller's 1979 address as first President of the Academy:

> Behavior medicine is an interdisciplinary field concerned with the integration of biomedical and behavioral [and I want to add *social*] knowledge relevant to health and disease . . .

> Behavioral medicine involves the integration of the relevant components of epidemiology, anthropology, sociology, psychology, physiology, pharmacology, neuroanatomy, endocrinology, immunology, and the various branches of medicine as well as related professions such as dentistry, nursing, and social work . . . (Miller, 1981).

Now, years later, we add to this integration between biomedical and social/behavioral knowledge a new dimension: aging. That is, by involving scholarship from the National Institute on Aging (NIA), we are adding a process-oriented or dynamic dimension. We are examining selected aspects of Neal Miller's concerns, including the immunological, the cognitive, and the physiological—but we shall now be examining them in a new light, as components of health, behavior, and aging. Thus we are looking at behavioral medicine as involving the aging of human beings over time. And we are looking at aging as

1

"biopsychosocial," that is, as a set of biomedical, behavioral, and social processes that interact and influence one another over time. In short, we are attempting here to specify and clarify how aging operates as the dynamic dimension in the continuing interplay between health and behavior. From our several perspectives, all of us here hope to share our understanding of what is known, take inventory of what is currently under study, and outline research agendas for the future in this increasingly integrated area.

As a social scientist, I want to set the stage for these multidisciplinary discussions by first stating the principles with which I approach our common task, and then outlining three perspectives on aging that may be useful in guiding our joint endeavors.

First, the principles:

- Aging is mutifaceted, consisting of social and psychological as well as biological processes.
- Aging is not entirely fixed for all time, but varies with social structure and social change.
- And, as a corollary, because aging is not immutable, it is subject to a degree of social and behavioral as well as biomedical modification and intervention.

To repeat: Aging is not entirely immutable, but changes as society changes, which means that aging is amenable to social control. Thus aging is centrally related to the concerns of behavioral medicine.

I suppose that these prinicples seem more self-evident to us social and behavioral scientists than to the biomedical scientists among us. It is we who stress the variability in the aging processes: While some people lead long, healthy, effective, and fulfilling lives, other people succumb early to ill health, loneliness, and withdrawal from affairs. It is we social and behavioral scientists who adduce the life-style examples of the Samoans who age differently when they migrate to Hawaii, and still more differently when they migrate to California (as shown in ongoing research by Ivan Pawson). While we emphasize the conditions of social and cultural variability in aging, the biomedical scientists are more likely to emphasize species-specific universals in the aging process. Yet, members of the human species do not grow old in laboratories. And universal aging processes must be gleaned, not from studies of any single cohort, but from many cohorts under the most widely varying social and temporal conditions.

I shall attempt to elucidate these principles during the three brief sections of this chapter, which are devoted to three biopsychosocial perspectives on aging:

1. *A cross-section perspective*, which describes and compares older people with younger people at a given period of time. This perspective is useful for describing age differences and current interactions among people who

differ in age. But if we want to understand the dynamic processes through which these age differences arise, the other two perspectives are essential;

2. *a life-course perspective*, which examines biomedical and psychosocial processes as they continually influence one another from birth to death; and

3. *a cohort perspective*, which examines how these aging processes respond to social change, so that cohorts of people who are growing old today age differently from cohorts who grew old in the past and from those who will grow old in the future.

The papers in this volume, like the discussions at the conference, present much scientific and often technical information about aging. It may help you, as it helps me, to remember that such information can usefully be viewed from each of these three perspectives—with widely differing interpretations and implications (Riley, 1973; 1985).

THE CROSS-SECTION PERSPECTIVE

The cross-section perspective on biopsychosocial aging is the familiar approach to which most research has so far been devoted. This perspective is highly useful but is also, if misused, potentially highly misleading.

The usefulness of observing age differences by comparing older with younger people at a given time can be illustrated from many current studies.[1] For example, in a cross-section study of healthy people aged 50 to 80, Howard Leventhal found few age differences in cognitive representations of various illnesses (such as reported symptoms, causes, consequences, treatments), but significant age differences in the associated emotions. Thus anger generated by the "cancer" label decreases by age, as do fear and shame associated with alcoholism, arthritis, and senility, age differences which could have implications for therapy or for family relations, for example, where the significant actors differ in age. But why these age differences? Leventhal's study begins to lead into life-course explanations (my second perspective) by noting that emotional upsets may be offset by the older person's prior experience with successful coping with such problems. (As you can see, every cross-section example leads further into the questions examined from the other two perspectives: How does a person develop particular coping strategies over the life course? How do such strategies aid in managing the emotional, if not the physiological, manifestations of disease? . . .)

---

[1]Studies for which no reference is cited, most of them by Academy members, are under way in the Behavioral Sciences Research program at NIA.

Another example of cross-sectional age differences refers to disease-related attitudes of the nursing staff in a general hospital (Ciliberto, Levin, & Arluke, 1981). When compared with younger persons with identical neuropsychiatric symptoms, older persons are more likely to be defined by these nurses as having organic brain syndrome, more likely to be given a poor prognosis for recovery, and more likely to be given palliative rather than interventionist treatment. Thus the age of the patient can influence clinical decisions that affect treatment.

A related age difference is discussed by Williams and Hadler (1983) who argue for de-emphasizing a disease-specific focus in the care of older, in contrast to younger, patients. Since the elderly typically present with multiple chronic diseases, these authors urge that a major goal should be to improve patient function and satisfaction, not merely to attempt a cure of underlying single diseases (such as incontinence, low back pain, or geriatric hand function). Along similar lines, Manton (1982) argues that for the elderly both prevention and therapy should focus not on single diseases, but on integrated approaches to multiple diseases.

Apart from many such studies of health attitudes and behaviors, a large body of current research points to age differences in personal characteristics (such as abilities, attitudes, education, or income) as well as to age differences in sheer numbers. Every day we hear new statistics on the mounting numbers of older people, with the population proportions of those 65 or older estimated to rise from 11% in 1980 (25.7 million people) to a possible 21% by 2030 (64.6 million people). The fastest growing segment of all are the "oldest old," those 85 or older. Cross-section views of the numbers and kinds of people in the several age strata are necessary for understanding the societal *context* affecting health and illness. As their mounting numbers outstrip the social roles and opportunities available to them, older people are under increasing pressure to withdraw from work and other useful activities, to allow their skills to atrophy, to define themselves as incompetent, and often to become mentally or physically ill.

However, all such cross-section descriptions, essential as they are for describing the status of older people in relation to younger people today, can also lead to a serious fallacy, what I call the "life-course fallacy," if age differences are erroneously interpreted as describing the aging process. Just consider the following stereotypes which, though using cross-section data for evidence, simply assert that aging—that is, the process of growing older—is subject to inevitable and universal decline:

- It was long believed that, because of aging, intelligence peaks in the second decade of life and then steadily declines.
- Similar universal and inevitable aging declines are presumed to affect sensation, perception, and the ability to react quickly to stimuli.
- Still accepted without question in medical textbooks are the classic diagrams, developed years ago by my colleague, Nathan Shock, which show a nearly

linear decrease from age 30 to age 80 in such functions as nerve conduction velocity, heart output, and maximum breathing capacity (Shock, 1976).

All such stereotypes of universal and inevitable decline, when derived from cross-section studies, are open to question. We all know that everyone dies. We know that certain biological declines must precede death in human beings, as they do in animals. But the nature and timing of particular declines cannot be accepted uncritically from the cross-section stereotypes, and many of these stereotypes are at last being subjected to serious scrutiny. Some stereotypes, like the decline in intelligence, have been demonstrated to result from fallacious interpretation of cohort differences—arising simply because the more recent cohorts are markedly better educated than were their predecessors. Other stereotypes have been traced, not to biological aging but to diminished social contacts, loss of employment, reduced sense of personal control, or inadequate health care. New questions are continually being raised about the effects of age as distinct from the effects of particular diseases or psychological states. Thus in current studies of dementia, using the PET scan, my colleague at the National Institute on Aging, Stanley I. Rapoport, has been able to negate earlier findings of a correlation between age and glucose metabolism in the brain (under resting conditions)—apparently the earlier studies did not screen the subjects for age-associated diseases. Or in studies of stress by Judith Rodin, which she describes in a later chapter of this volume, early findings show that the stress reactions of different types of immune cells are related more to functional than to chronological age.

Still other stereotypes of inevitable aging decline are being challenged through experiments demonstrating that certain decrements of old age can often be restored or reversed through social interventions. Thus research by P. Baltes and Willis (1982) shows that intellectual decline with aging (when it occurs) can often be slowed or reversed with opportunities for added practice, with instructions about strategies for approaching the problem and with incentives that increase motivation and attention. Rodin, M. Baltes, and others have shown that many serious disabilities, even when experienced in nursing homes, can be reduced by social regimens that provide retraining or reward activity and independence (Rodin, 1980; Baltes, 1982). Even slowed reaction time in performing psychomotor tasks, long attributed to aging losses in central nervous system functioning, seems also to be affected by psychosocial factors (such as unclear contingencies, uncertain feedback, over-eagerness to avoid mistakes). Reports from experiments by Alan Baron at the University of Wisconsin show that, following carefully designed training sessions, older subjects can effectively reverse deficits in the performance of tasks under time pressure.

Thus the evidence is accumulating that the aging process is to a degree variable and subject to improvement through social intervention (one of my principles). Nevertheless, the stereotypes of inevitable aging decline remain persistent and widespread. Such stereotypes are dangerous because they can become self-fulfilling prophecies. At one extreme, all the problems and behaviors of old age become reinterpreted as illnesses, with a mandate to biomedical researchers to find some cure or treatment (this phenomenon has been called the "accidental medicalization of old age"—Arluke & Peterson, 1981). Alternatively, at the other extreme, all of the diseases and disabilities of old age are reinterpreted as "normal aging" and given little serious medical attention. Thus many physicians, because they continue to look on aging as a process of inevitable deterioration (Coe & Brehm, 1972), spend less time in office visits with older patients than with younger ones (Kane, Solomon, Beck, Keeler, & Kane, 1980), and give them less elaborate and drastic treatment (DeVita, 1980). Old people themselves also tend to accept this negative stereotype, to take their aches and pains for granted, and to seek palliative rather than preventive or corrective treatment (Riley, Foner, Moore, Hess, & Roth, 1968). As Leventhal's study shows, old people unlike younger people tend to attribute to old age the common symptom of fatigue, rather than seeking medical help for some potentially underlying disease that might be treatable.

Clearly, then, the cross-section perspective on aging as a process gives incomplete and often misleading findings. Much further examination is needed from the dynamic perspectives in order to understand the nature of the individual aging processes over the life course and the differing patterns of aging among successive cohorts of individuals as society changes. Let me leave this cross-section perspective with a cautionary note: False stereotypes of inevitable and universal aging decline die hard. Though I came to the National Institutes of Health expecting to stimulate new and dynamic examination of aging as a process, all too often I still find myself in a Nietzschean nightmare of endlessly fighting the same old false cross-sectional stereotypes.

THE LIFE-COURSE PERSPECTIVE

Turning now to the second perspective, the life-course perspective (I shall have less to say about the two dynamic perspectives, since less has yet been accomplished), here we seek to understand how biomedical and psychosocial aging processes continually influence one another from birth to death. Just as we need to dispel false stereotypes of the complete immutability of old age, we need also to enlarge scientific understanding of the variabilities in the aging process, and to identify particular mechanisms and conditions that can optimize that process— that can prevent or reverse many of the currently associated disabilities.

To conceptualize this perspective, I like to think of the aging of an individual as represented by a diagonal bar (see Figure 1.1) that moves upward with aging, but also horizontally with historical time. As people age, they change socially and psychologically as well as biologically; they accumulate knowledge, attitudes, and experiences; they move through social roles in family, school, and

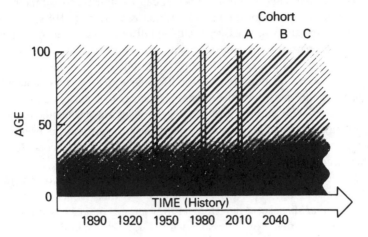

FIGURE 1.1.   The age stratification system: A schematic view.

work in the changing society. Of course, each bar in my schematic representation is not unitary, but consists of all the diverse strands in the aging process. Thus we must take into account:

- Biological aging processes (neural, immunological, endocrine, and other physiological changes with aging);
- Cognitive and biopsychologial aging processes (change or constancy in intellectual or sensori-motor functioning);
- Attitudinal and motivational aging processes (change or constancy in self-esteem, personal control, coping, maintaining a sense of personal identity); and
- Social aging processes (not only reactions to "events" but also growing older within particular roles, actively shaping these roles, relating to and interacting with significant other people).

One task before us is to consider how all of these strands, themselves changing with age, interact with one another as a person grows older; and how a change in any one strand creates feedback loops in the others. This is hardly a simple task! But here, I believe, lies the challenge and the opportunity for fresh insights.

Strangely enough, little work has yet been done on biopsychosocial aging from a life-course perspective. A case in point is research on stress. The Institute of Medicine's Committee on Stress delved deeply into the relationships among four elements: environmental stressors, their antecedents, the consequent health outcomes, and the causal connections among them. Yet, as members of that

Committee, Beatrix Hamburg and I had practically no success in convincing the other members that each of these elements can be influenced by their place in the aging process. The published report (Elliott & Eisdorfer, 1982) makes clear that, with rare exceptions, stress in health and disease has not been studied from a life-course perspective, as stress affects, and is affected by, social, psychological and biological processes of aging. Still remaining are the many dynamic questions: questions of ordering over the life course of stressful events and their consequences; and questions of how the sequences of stressors and health outcomes are linked with the concurrent and accompanying age-related changes (cf. Riley, 1983a). For example, does bereavement have different consequences in mid-life when accompanied by responsibilities of family and work than in late life when accompanied with frailty and living alone?

Nevertheless, important beginnings have been made in life-course studies of biopsychosocial aging, in particular by members of this Academy. With respect to cardiovascular disease, Alan Herd (1982) among others has pointed to the impact of aging on many of the associated risk factors, including dissatisfaction with interpersonal relations, job demands beyond a person's control, or sudden severe sense of loss. Herd notes that a few studies have found coronary-prone behavior patterns to be more widespread among middle-aged than among older subjects and coping techniques to shift from active to passive as people grow old. Yet much remains on the agenda here for us biomedical and social/behavioral scientists who are concerned with the aging process. If Pattern A is a precursor to coronary heart disease, when does the pattern first manifest itself? Can its origins be traced to early life experiences? To what extent do the consequences accumulate with aging? If, indeed, the pattern shifts as people grow older, what are the nature and the conditions of such shifts? With respect to the immune system, Robert Ader (1981) among others points out that certain behavioral factors believed to modulate immunologic reactivity (e.g., factors associated with sleeplessness, nutritional disorders, or bereavement) are vulnerable to aging, as is the immune system itself. (Several chapters in this volume, as well as much of the discussion at the conference, build on Ader's promising work.)

How health or disease translate into functioning involves psychosocial issues of social context, social support, definitions of illness, and ability to cope (as George Maddox notes in a later chapter). All too little attention is paid to social contexts. Yet, specific characteristics of the work role have been shown by Melvin Kohn and colleagues, as well as by other researchers, to have striking effects on the aging process. Thus complexity of the job, lack of routinization, and freedom from close supervision can, as people grow older, improve their intellectual functioning and their mental (and perhaps ultimately their physical) well-being (Kohn & Schooler, 1983; Kahn, Lawler, & Seashore, 1981).

Also still on our research agenda are studies of life-course styles of coping with "daily hassles" at work or in the family—how and when and under what circumstances do coping styles develop and change as people grow older? And what about social support, which appears from the studies of Cobb (1979), House and Robbins (1983), and others to protect against disabling conditions, accelerate recovery, or facilitate compliance with prescribed regimens? A cross-section analysis by Robert Kahn is showing that the size of social support networks, typically smaller for men than for women, tends to decrease by age. But what would be learned about changes in nature and effectiveness of social supports if the same individuals were followed longitudinally over time? More generally, what would be learned if differing life-course patterns, the improving as well as the deteriorating, were compared and analyzed by multivariate techniques, instead of being aggregated into a single modal statistic?

Such beginnings seem sufficient to open significant topics for research from the life-course perspective. Certainly they are sufficient to emphasize my principle that aging consists of interdependent psychological and social as well as biological processes, and to warrant further attention to the conditions engendering variability and mutability in the ways that people grow old.

THE COHORT PERSPECTIVE

This variability of the aging process, and the conditions under which the process is mutable, can be probed not only by tracing the lives of individuals who are growing old today, but also by comparing cohorts of individuals who grow old under differing historical and future conditions. This brings us to my third and final perspective, the cohort perspective, which examines the aging process as it is responsive to social change.

In considering all three of these perspectives, it is often helpful to imagine (as in Figure 1.1) a series of diagonal bars within a space bounded on its vertical axis by years of age (from 0 to 100 or so) and on its horizontal axis by historical time (as from 1900 to 2000 and later). Each diagonal bar (the life-course perspective) represents an individual (or cohort of individuals born at the same time) who is aging—moving upward with aging and across time as society is changing. The series of diagonal bars (the cohort perspective) represents the succession of cohorts, as new cohorts of people are continually being born, aging from birth to death, and moving through historical time. The cross-section perspective, then, represents a vertical slice through all of these diagonal bars. Clearly, when we compare older with younger people we are studying differences not only in age, but also in the differing cohorts to which these people belong—hence the potential life-course fallacy.

For the cohort perspective this schematic representation is useful because it forces us to keep in mind that each cohort cuts off a unique segment of historical time—confronts its own particular sequence of social and environmental events and changes. Members of United States cohorts who are old today were born early in this century, grew up prior to the discoveries of antibiotics or the polio vaccine, and experienced two World Wars and the Great Depression. These people cannot have aged in precisely the same way as cohorts who lived in earlier times, or as those cohorts now in their younger years who will grow old in the future.

This general recognition that aging is mutable, that people in different cohorts age in different ways, is becoming increasingly accepted by students of aging (Riley, Abeles, & Teitelbaum, 1982), although the links between historical changes and aging processes are barely beginning to be studied. From existing studies it is now clear that members of cohorts already old differ markedly from those in cohorts not yet old in many critical respects that can influence health and functioning: diet, exercise, standard of living, education, work history, medical care, and experience with chronic vs. acute diseases. Successive cohorts of young people are on the average taller than their parents, and successive cohorts of young women start to menstruate at younger ages.

Perhaps most striking of all the cohort differences are the unprecedented increases in longevity (over two-thirds of the world's improvement in longevity from prehistoric times until the present has taken place in the brief period since 1900—Preston, 1976). Not until the 1983 meetings of the American Association for the Advancement of Science were the recent and entirely unpredicted mortality declines among the very old reported (from NIA-supported work by Eileen Crimmins, Kenneth Manton, Ira Rosenwaike, and others). These increases in longevity, combined with the baby-boom cohorts, have produced undreamed-of numbers of older people, especially at the oldest ages where by 1983 (at age 85+) women outnumbered men by 241 to 100! Massive questions are raised by these changes about the place of older people in society, as demands of work life are increasingly ambiguous, and as family life is transformed by added generations and new step-kin relations (Riley, 1983b). In particular, two critical questions, though now widely discussed, remain largely unanswered: the relation to health and the relation to death. As the numbers of old people mount, will the added years increase the proportion who are disabled and dependent? Or will the majority of older people remain reasonably healthy and able to function reasonably well, with death simply postponed until a still-older age? (Who at the beginning of this century could have dreamed that by 1980 two-thirds of all deaths would occur after age 65?—Brody and Brock, 1985.)

With regard to the health of future cohorts of older people, studies of risk factors are beginning to offer some clues—at a time when half of U.S. deaths are being attributed to behavioral and life-style factors. Cigarette smoking, the most deadly of the health risk factors, provides one example of how life-preserving behaviors can be responsive to changes in society (Riley, 1981; U.S. Department of Health and Human Services, 1981). Over the past decades each successive cohort of adult males in the United States—presumably responsive to the Surgeon General's warnings—has been less likely than its predecessors to smoke cigarettes. For women, however, the proportions who smoked increased from cohort to cohort—in line with the "liberation" of women—up until the health warnings of the mid-1960s; since then, the most recent cohorts of women are beginning to follow the declining pattern. Thus predictably, the death rates attributable to smoking, currently increasing for women, can be expected to decline as these more recent cohorts grow older.

Another study which suggests that more recent cohorts are increasingly aware of their own future health comes from the Framingham Heart Study, where the lives of some 1,600 married couples have been traced for many years. Recently, a parallel study has been made of their offspring (Feinlieb, 1975), comparing the offspring cohorts today with the cohorts of their parents 22 years ago when they were approximately the same ages. The age-controlled differences between these two cohorts in three of the major risk factors in coronary heart disease are striking: The offspring, as compared with their parents, show lower blood pressure, lower serum cholesterol, and less cigarette smoking. These differences suggest that the cohorts who will be old in the future may be healthier, at least in certain respects, than cohorts already old today—that old age diseases and disabilities may be postponed.

Whatever the health of older people of the future, the sheer increases in numbers guarantee that care for the old in the last months of life will be enormously costly both to society and to the old people themselves and to their families. (It has been estimated that nearly one third of total Medicare expenditure is made during the terminal year of life.) There will be ethical questions of triage in the allotting of medical care. Even more poignant, there will increasingly be questions of how long to sustain life for those elderly who are moribund and senescent. As medical advances allow organic life to be prolonged long after behavioral life has ended, the relevant knowledge base must come from students of behavioral medicine. Morris Abrams, who chaired the President's Commission on Ethical Problems in Biomedical and Behavioral Research, states that this is not an issue for the lawyers (*New York Times*, June 5, 1983). A critical review of the burgeoning and often confusing social science literature on dying by John Riley (1983) points clearly to problems of euthanasia for the oncoming cohorts of older people. Manton (1982) makes the case that the unanticipated mortality reductions at the oldest ages, occurring in the 1960s and 1970s, point to entirely new and not yet understood biological and social mechanisms now influencing the aging process. Such problems can be uniquely addressed by this Academy.

All such dramatic cohort differences show emphatically that we cannot understand old age as it is today or will be in the future by relying on existing studies of people who were old in the recent past. In this sense, and quite apart from disease, I myself try to avoid the expression "normal" aging. What seems "normal" may mean merely "cohort-centric," that is, thinking of aging generally as we have experienced it in our own particular cohorts.

In sum, the agenda set by this conference transcends both aging and behavioral medicine per se. Aging is the time dimension along which all biological, psychological, and social processes of concern to us are moving. We cannot understand aging without examining the interaction between behavior and health. By the same token, we cannot understand behavioral medicine—the mechanisms linking behavior and health—without regard to the process-oriented aspects of individual aging and the impact of social change on these aging processes. Both the life-course and the cohort perspectives are needed.

This volume points to the remarkable opportunity for multidisciplinary interchange on the many questions that will emerge—such questions, for example, as those proposed earlier by Ader (1981) for examining the relation of behavior to the immune system:

- What hormonal changes accompany psychologically induced immunologic changes, and how are these influenced by aging?
- What are the connections between the brain and the immune system that enable an exchange of information, and how are these influenced by aging?
- Can behavioral modification or social interventions affect the self-regulation of immunologic reactivity, and how is this potential influenced by aging?

Or more generally, we shall be discussing such questions as:

- How do the biological and psychosocial aging processes link up?
- Under what conditions and to what extent can age-related decrements be slowed or reversed?
- What light is cast by our current knowledge of biopsychosocial aging on how people are likely to age in the future?
- How can the relatively vigorous health, effective functioning, and productivity of the middle years be extended into the later years?

This is a heady agenda. The tone was set by David Hamburg, the Academy's second President, whose Institute of Medicine initiative was reported earlier under the title: *Health and Behavior: Frontiers of Research in the Biobehavioral Sciences* (Hamburg, Elliott, & Parron, 1982). I believe that these new papers, and the subsequent work they should engender, will advance these frontiers immeasurably and will do so through the incorporation of aging—the neglected dynamic dimension of behavioral medicine research. Through this volume, we are seeking new insights and new research questions.

ACKNOWLEDGMENTS

Keynote address, Annual Conference of the Academy for Behavioral Medicine Research, Reston, Virginia, June 5, 1983. For helpful comments on earlier versions of the manuscript, the author is indebted to Margret Baltes, Paul Baltes, Alan Baron, Eileen Crimmins, Kenneth Manton, Stanley Rapoport, and other colleagues at the National Institute on Aging, as well as to her long-time collaborator, John W. Riley, Jr.

REFERENCES

Ader, R. (1981, November). *Health, behavior, and aging: Research needs.* Paper presented to the Gerontological Society of America, Toronto, Canada.

Arluke, A., & Peterson, J. (1981). Accidental medicalization of old age and its social control implications. In C. L. Fry (Ed.), *Dimensions: Aging, culture, and health* (pp. 271–284). New York: J. F. Bergin Publishers.

Baltes, M. M. (1982). Environmental factors in dependency among nursing home residents: A social ecology analysis. In A. T. Wills (Ed.), *Basic processes in helping relationships.* New York: Academic Press.

Baltes, P. B., & Willis, S. L. (1982). Plasticity and enhancement of intellectual functioning in old age. In F. I. M. Craik & S. E. Trehub (Eds.), *Aging and cognitive processes.* New York: Plenum Press.

Brody, J. A., & Brock, D. B. (1985). Epidemiological and statistical characteristics of the United States' elderly population. In C. Finch & E. Schneider (Eds.), *Handbook of the biology of aging* (rev. ed. pp. 3–26). New York: Van Nostrand Reinhold.

Ciliberto, D. J., Levin, J., & Arluke, A. (1981). Nurses' diagnostic stereotyping of the elderly: The case of organic brain syndrome. *Research on Aging, 3*(3), 299–310.

Cobb, S. (1979). Social support and health through the life course. In M. W. Riley (Ed.), *Aging from birth to death: Interdisciplinary perspectives* (pp. 93–106). Boulder, CO: Westview Press.

Coe, R. M., & Brehm, H. P. (1972). *Preventive health care for adults: A study of medical practice.* New Haven, CT: Yale University Press.

DeVita, V. T. (1980). *Statement before the Select Committee on Aging.* House of Representatives, September 26, 1980. Communications Publication No. 96–275.

Elliott, G. R., & Eisdorfer, C. (Eds.). (1982). *Stress and human health: Analysis and implications of research.* New York: Springer Publishing Company.

Feinleib, M. (1975). The Framingham offspring study: Design and preliminary data. *Preventive Medicine, 4,* 518–525.

Hamburg, D. A., Elliott, G. R., & Parron, D. L. (1982). *Health and behavior: Frontiers of research in the biobehavioral sciences.* Washington, D.C.: National Academy Press.

Herd, J. A. (1982, January). *Behavioral influences on cardiovascular disease.* Paper presented to the AAAS III Symposium on Aging from Birth to Death III: Biosocial Perspectives.

House, J. S., & Robbins, C. (1983). Age, psychosocial stress, and health. In M. W. Riley, B. B. Hess, & K. Bond (Eds.), *Aging in society: Selected reviews of recent research* (pp. 175–197). Hillsdale, NJ: Lawrence Erlbaum Associates.

Kahn, R., Lawler III, E., & Seashore, S. (Eds.). (1981). *Work and health.* New York: John Wiley and Sons.

Kane, R., Solomon, D., Beck, J., Keeler, E., & Kane, R. (1980). The future need for geriatric manpower in the United States. *New England Journal of Medicine, 302,* 1327–1332.

Kohn, M., & Schooler, C. (1983). *Work and personality: An inquiry into the impact of social stratification.* Norwood, NJ: Ablex Press.

Manton, K. J. (1982). Changing concepts of morbidity and mortality in the elderly population. *Milbank Memorial Fund Quarterly, 60,* 183–244.

Miller, N. E. (1981). An overview of behavioral medicine: Opportunities and dangers. In S. M. Weiss, J. A. Herd, & B. H. Fox (Eds.), *Perspectives on behavioral medicine* (pp. 3–22). New York: Academic Press.

Preston, S. H. (1976). *Mortality patterns in national populations: With special reference to recorded causes of death.* New York: Academic Press.

Riley, J. W., Jr. (1983). Dying and the meanings of death: Sociological inquiries. *Annual Review of Sociology, 9,* 191–216.

Riley, M. W. (1973). Aging and cohort succession: Interpretations and misinterpretations. *The Public Opinion Quarterly, 37,* 35–49.

Riley, M. W. (1981). Health behavior of older people: Toward a new paradigm. In D. L. Parron, F. Solomon, & J. Rodin (Eds.), *Health, behavior and aging* (pp. 25–39). Washington, DC: National Academy Press.

Riley, M. W. (1983a). Cancer and the life course. In R. Yancik, P. P. Carbone, W. P. Patterson, K. Steel, & W. D. Terry, (Eds.), *Prevention and treatment of cancer in the elderly* (pp. 25–32). New York: Raven Press.

Riley, M. W. (1983b). The family in an aging society: A matrix of latent relationships. *Journal of Family Issues, 4*, 439–454.

Riley, M. W. (1985). Age strata in social systems. In R. H. Binstock & E. Shanas (Eds.), *Handbook on aging and social sciences* (rev. ed., pp. 369–411). New York: Van Nostrand Reinhold.

Riley, M. W., Abeles, R. P., & Teitelbaum, M. S. (Eds.). (1982). *Aging from birth to death, Volume II: Sociotemporal perspectives*. Boulder, CO: Westview Press.

Riley, M. W., Foner, A., Moore, M. E., Hess, B., & Roth, B. (1968). *Aging and society, Volume I: An inventory of research findings*. New York: Sage.

Rodin, J. (1980). Managing the stress of aging: The role of control and coping. In S. Levine & H. Ursin (Eds.), *Coping and health*. New York: Plenum.

Shock, N. W. (1976). System Integration. In C. E. Finch & L. Hayflick (Eds.), *Handbook of the biology of aging* (pp. 639–665). New York: Van Nostrand Reinhold.

U.S. Dept. of Health and Human Services. (1981). *Health: United States 1981*. Hyattsville, MD: DHHS Publication No. (PHS) 82–1232, National Center for Health Statistics.

Williams, M. E., & Hadler, N. M. (1983, June). Sounding board: The illness as the focus of geriatric medicine. *New England Journal of Medicine, 308*, 1357–1359.

2

PSYCHOSOCIAL PERSPECTIVES ON AGING

George L. Maddox
Duke University

Leonard Silk, a science writer who covers economics for *The New York Times*, not long ago listened for several days to a group of scientists discussing various aspects of aging processes. Scientists, he observed, love to dissect and reduce problems to the level at which they are intellectually comfortable but demonstrate little affection for putting the pieces back together. Mr. Silk, originally trained as an academic, understood but regretted the intellectual, political, and practical forces which impel scientists to specialize and to focus on a narrow range of problems which they believe they can solve with available disciplinary theory and methods. He would, therefore, be pleased to note the existence of the Academy of Behavioral Medicine Research (ABMR), the legislatively mandated commitment of the National Institute on Aging (NIA) to multidisciplinary research, and the interest of NIA and the Institute of Medicine in promoting discussion of interrelationships among health, behavior, and aging.

The disentanglement of physiological functioning and change which are primary to developmental process, on the one hand, from functioning and change which are secondary to disease or to factors exogenous to organisms, on the other hand, is a complex but fundamental task. It is these secondary and exogenous factors which are substantially the province of the psychosocial sciences and potentially provide the groundwork for interdisciplinary scientific discussion.

My objectives in beginning the discussion are modest. In my view, a broad, systematic agenda for interdisciplinary research among physiological and psychosocial scientists would be premature at this time. It is enough to review some key issues in the perspectives of behavioral medicine, of an older tradition of social medicine, and of the study of aging and to identify some intersections of scientific interests. In conclusion, several suggestions for research will be proposed. Particular attention will be given to contemporary scientific interest in stress—its etiology, correlates, consequences, and probable amelioration—and to the emergence of experimental social gerontology. Both these developments illustrate the intersection of research on neuroendocrine and social systems and the physiological systems (as illustrated by the neuroendoctrinal system (for a full review see Finch, 1977, 1985).

BEHAVIORAL MEDICINE: A NEW PERSPECTIVE

Neal Miller (1981) has noted a new interest expressed as *behavioral medicine* in response to increased awareness of biomedical issues with an obvious and large behavioral component. The observed pattern of disease has changed dramatically in the second half of this century. Morbidity and mortality patterns in contemporary industrial society that preoccupy health professionals currently reflect chronic rather than acute disease processes. Since the incidence and prevalence of chronic conditions are known to increase with chronological age, the aging of populations promises continuing challenges for biomedical scientists and health professionals which cannot be ignored. At the heart of these challenges, Miller correctly perceives, is what David Mechanic has called the *nonspecificity* of the dominant patterns of disease currently observed: Nonspecificity refers to the relative absence of single-factor etiology, predictable natural course, and definitive intervention as illustrated by heart disease, cancer, mental illness, and substance abuse. Heart disease and cancer are medical problems with substantial behavioral—and one might add *social*—components quite possibly in regard to etiology and certainly in regard to the course of these conditions and their management. Some mental illness, affect disorders, and substance abuse may even be usefully conceived as essentially behavioral and social disorders with medical concomitants. Chronic disease processes and related illness and responses to illness simply will not reduce to biological explanations alone.

In the past decade the concept of risk has added an interesting new dimension to the study of chronic disease. Learned, socially induced and reinforced behavior and lifestyles have been implicated in explaining the incidence and course of a variety of chronic disease processes. These risks are exogenous to but are expressed through biological systems. It follows that the reduction of risky behavior and lifestyles through social learning and reinforcement can enhance biological functioning and survival (Wiley & Comacho, 1980).

Scientists with interest in behavioral medicine have documented pioneering observations about the behavioral components in the etiology, course, and management of chronic disease (Weiss, Herd, & Fox, 1981; Hine, Carson, Maddox, Thompson, & Williams, 1983). These contributions do not require repetition here. What may warrant comment are parallel, complementary developments in social medicine and in the study of aging. In behavioral medicine, the primary focus is on the individual. In social medicine, the primary focus is on interpersonal interaction, groups, populations, and environments. Research on aging has historically been decidedly multidisciplinary in its emphasis on individuals, social systems, and the interaction of individuals and environments.

SOCIAL MEDICINE

Some medical historians have proposed that medicine is ultimately a social science (e.g., McKeown, 1965). This conclusion reflects the documentation that, historically, major changes in the health status and survival of populations are more adequately attributed to changes in community hygiene, stability and distribution of food supply, and lifestyle than to advances in biomedical science (for recent statements see Walker, 1983, and Fuchs, 1983). Patterns of morbidity and mortality reflect the embeddedness of individuals in social and cultural contexts which are differentially benign or hostile to survival and well-being. Observed differences in the life expectancy of different populations historically and currently are substantial with average life expectancy varying by more than two decades between populations in more or less developed nations (Siegel, 1981; Myers, 1982). Currently, in five countries of the world, average life expectancy at birth is less than 40 years. In more developed countries, average life expectancy at birth is 68.4 years for males and 75.7 years for females. In contrast, in less developed countries the comparable life expectancies are 54.2 and 56 years. In the next two decades, average life expectancy at birth is predicted to increase for males and females in more developed countries by about two years and in less developed countries by about seven years. The observed differences and predicted changes are better explained causally by social than by biological factors.

Further, socioeconomic status has been and remains currently a powerful predictor of different patterns of morbidity, mortality, and longevity (Syme & Berkman, 1976; Wiley & Comacho, 1980). Among the risk factors detrimental to health, survival, and well-being, factors such as impoverishment, ignorance, and social disorganization warrant the kinds of attention more likely to be given currently to smoking, cholesterol, inactivity, and stress. All of these negative factors are related to lower socioeconomic status. Or put another way, the popular statements of risks associated with unhealthy lifestyles and behavior have a demonstrable association with the impoverishment and lack of education which are typically used to index lower socioeconomic status. For this reason, discussions of risk factors and their modification without discussion of societal stratification and related resource allocation are naïve if not perversely negligent.

The perspective of social medicine, with its strong ties to epidemiology and demography, is essentially multivariate and contextual, and complements the relatively individualistic perspective of behavioral medicine. From the perspective of social medicine, the biological functioning of individuals (hosts) and their responses to noxious agents are never properly understood apart from the physical and sociocultural context within which individuals function. The late John Cassel (1976) was particularly articulate in making a case for social epidemiology in the context of social medicine, especially in his broadening of the definition of *noxious agents* to include the relevance for health and illness of social factors such as crowding, rapid social change, cultural disorganization, social isolation, and the absence of essential social support. Cassel argued that social factors, and particularly social support by kith and kin, are potentially preventative and certainly ameliorative factors for individuals responding to possibly stressful events. This idea is a major contribution to conceptualizing needed research on stress and its management. He anticipated correctly that the biological mechanisms through which stress modification worked were three of the systems of interest to behavioral medicine—the central nervous system, the endocrine system, and the immune system. One notes with interest that the literature of behavioral medicine identifies social contexts and support as both causal and mediating in stress and variable in response to stress and, in the process, acknowledges a fourth system—the social system. Social systems affect health and illness and responses of individuals and social groups to them (see, Weksler, 1981).

Rudolf Moos (1974, 1980) has made the case for a social ecological perspective in research on health and illness in a particularly interesting way. Environmental factors generally and factors in the immediate contexts of behavior (milieus) have treatment effects. He has illustrated the usefulness of this perspective in studying families, organizations, clinics, and communities. Experimental scientists typically illustrate their understanding of potentially confounding environmental effects by rigid control of contextual factors. Such control in human research in natural context is not acceptable and scientists must settle for quasi-experiments. In any case, all scientists recognize the potential importance of exogenous, contextual factors in research on human beings. The tendency among biological scientists is to control variables exogenous to individuals rather than to treat them as experimental variables.

AGING

The awareness that aging can be and is associated with personal and social problems is ancient as is the awareness that many of these problems are sociogenic, not just biogenic (Maddox & Wiley, 1976). The systematic scientific study of aging is more recent, stimulated in large part by evidence of the aging of populations worldwide, of the association of age with dependency, and of the high personal and social cost of responding to age-related dependency. A sense of social urgency has characterized research on aging, particularly in the past two decades, as the societal implications of population aging have become clearer. One does not have to be a scientist to understand the issues of income maintenance associated with an average of almost two decades of survival post-retirement. The recurrent crisis of Social Security and growing awareness of the societal costs of geriatric care are cases in point. One needs only to read the newspapers. Or one may consult middle-aged colleagues to get a sense of the high probability that just at the time when adults are longing for relief from dealing with dependent children, the issue of dependent parents arises. This new issue of parent caring which is competing with interest in child caring is not being made easier by the long-term and continuing trend toward employment outside the home among married women, historically the caregivers of society, and changes in the composition of families, in living arrangements and in inter-generational relationships (see Fuchs, 1983).

This palpable sense of social urgency ensured that the social scientific and behavioral issues of aging would be prominent and, along with biological aspects of aging, receive attention. In fact, in my experience, study of aging processes in the United States have, to an unusual degree, been multidisciplinary from the outset. This was distinctly the case in the creation of the Gerontological Society in 1945 with sections on biology, clinical medicine, behavioral and social sciences, and social research and practice. The early university-based research centers and their research programs were also multidisciplinary. These developments help to explain why, when the NIA was created, Congress was encouraged to mandate legislatively a multidisciplinary institute that specified the inclusion of behavioral and social scientific research. The first report of the NIA to Congress, outlining its research agenda, used as its point of departure three handbooks summarizing research by gerontological scientists on the biological (Finch & Hayflick, 1977), behavioral (Birren & Schaie, 1977), and social scientific (Binstock & Shanas, 1976) aspects of aging.

Matilda White Riley, first as a scholar and scientist and more recently in her leadership role as an associate director of the NIA, has been an articulate advocate for multidisciplinary research on aging generally and for the intersection of interests among biological, behavioral, and social scientists specifically. Her summary propositions about what we know about human aging capture succinctly and well the current consensus (see, e.g., Riley, 1981, 1983):

1. Aging is a psychosocial as well as biological process.
2. Aging processes are not fixed and immutable, but reflect sociocultural contexts and changes in those contexts.
3. Aging processes are subject to some degree of human intervention and control.

Each of these propositions warrants brief elaboration.

The Multidimensionality and Variability
of Interrelated Aging Processes

The human life span has limits, although biologists argue about what the outer limits might be under various circumstances. The now-famous demonstration by Nathan Shock that the function of all adult biological systems has a negative age-related slope promises that we will all be dead in the long run. This perspective has encouraged a view of human aging emphasizing inevitable biological decrement and invited a persistent confusion between aging and illness, which is associated with but not necessarily synonymous with aging. More recently, biological scientists have begun to consider whether and how both the age-intercept and slope of measured function of biological systems might be modified beneficially. Recent beneficial changes in cardiovascular morbidity and mortality in the United States, for example, certainly reflect changes in sociogenic risk factors, not simply changes in genetics and medical care (Walker, 1983). Similarly, increased average life expectancy in developing countries reflects primarily the same changes in environmental and lifestyle factors that produced the radically changed age compositions of developed societies during the last century.

Variance observed in human aging processes and in the experience of aging warrants more attention than it has been given. Elementary textbooks in statistics admonish students that measures of central tendencies should be accompanied by measures of variance. Variance in research populations can be an artifact of measurement error or sampling bias but can also reflect real differences. Years ago, in the Duke Longitudinal Studies, a colleague and I (Maddox & Douglass, 1973) noted that variance in a wide variety of behavioral and physiological indicators remained constant over time in the study population. Variation around the mean of a study population potentially has various explanations—errors in measurement, genetics, learned and socially reinforced individual differences in lifestyles, and differential access to essential goods and services. The persistent power of social class placement as a predictor of morbidity, mortality, functional capacity, and well-being cannot be easily missed in adult populations. If observed variance in age-related processes can be explained in part by social factors, one inevitably wonders about the modifiability of these factors and the effects of these modifications.

Comparative social research within and between populations as well as demographic research on the age, gender, and social status-specific life tables demonstrate significant variability in the aging of populations at a particular time as well as over time. Societies with different resources available and policies for different allocation of resources over the life course constitute natural experiments in the effects of social factors on human aging. The diseases that killed our ancestors are not the ones that kill us. Individuals in more or less developed nations today die on a different schedule and for different reasons. Moreover, biologists are ultimately no more likely than anyone else to equate well-being with survival. Individuals of precisely the same chronological age within and between societies can and do experience substantial differences in subjective and objective quality of life—in economic security, in availability of health care, in opportunities for self-fulfillment, and in life satisfaction. Biological intactness alone does not ensure personal and social well-being. And personal and social well-being can be achieved or maintained in the face of considerable biological decrements. In spite of the demonstrated association between aging and biological decrements that ensures that a large majority of persons 65 years of age and older will have at least one chronic illness, average older adults, certainly in developed nations, live out their lives with a very high level of functional competence and with personal satisfaction.

The dominant contemporary view of health does not equate health and well-being simply with the absence of disease or compromised biological functioning but with the capacity of individuals to function adequately as social beings. The National Center for Health Statistics (NCHS) regularly reports that 8 out of 10 persons 65 years of age and older have at least one chronic disease, but a much smaller proportion (an estimated 14/100) are unable to perform essential personal and social tasks (National Center for Health Statistics, 1983). The presence of disease does not determine automatically the degree of impairment, disability, or handicap experienced. How disease, if present, translates into functional impairment clearly involves psychosocial factors. A particularly good illustration of this is the ameliorative effect of learned styles of coping with life events and social support groups in facilitating the maintenance of impaired older persons in the community. Coping styles and social groups can and apparently do modify significantly and mediate stressful events (see Pearlin, Lieberman, Menaghan, & Mullan, 1981; House & Robbins, 1983; Wheaton, 1983).

The concept of *risk factor* also calls attention to the psychosocial aspects of health and illness. Relatively recent reports in Canada (Lalonde, 1974) and the United States (Surgeon General, U.S., 1979) estimate that lifestyle and behavioral factors explain a majority of the disease, impairments, disabilities, and handicaps observed. The factors specified are familiar—diet, drugs, exercise, stress, and health habits. As noted earlier, we would add to these factors sociogenic risks such as poverty, ignorance, and social isolation.

The consideration of aging processes is particularly relevant to the consideration of risk factors for several reasons. First, exposure to risk factors in the adult years interacting with adult lifestyles modifies the probability of disease and functional incapacity in later life (Wiley & Comacho, 1980). Second, a life-course view of the effects of exposure to risk suggests that reduction of exposure would, in the long run, make a contribution to the health and well-being of future cohorts of older persons. Third, the personal and social consequences of continuing to do business as usual in a society with a high prevalence of unhealthy behavior and lifestyles are very unattractive. The aging of the U.S. population continues at a rapid rate, and the oldest population category (those 85 years of age and over) continues to grow at the most rapid rate of all. The functional capacity of older individuals which would ensure maximal independence and autonomy is, therefore, a major concern. In the absence of definitive evidence, what is expected is a matter of considerable controversy (Fries, 1980; Schneider & Brody, 1983). The limited current evidence is not reassuring. In a special study of remaining active (functionally competent) years of life in Massachusetts, Katz and associates (1983) estimated that for persons aged 60–69, there were 16.5 years of life remaining on average, ten of which (61%) were active years. The estimate of survival and active years decreased monotonically with age. For those 85 years and older, average remaining years of life were 7.3 with 2.9 of these (40%) estimated to be active years.

Modifiability of Aging Processes

Riley's second proposition declares optimistically that aging processes are mutable and that change is at least partly a function of social factors and social change. Change in average life expectancy for populations has increased dramatically in this century, particularly in developed countries, largely as a consequence of improved control of environments. The point is often made that age-specific life expectancy at 75 or 85 has changed very little. But even here there is some evidence of small but steady increases (Siegel, 1980; Myers, 1982; NCHS, 1983). The probability of surviving to and beyond age 85 is increasing worldwide. In the United States, mortality rates of very old persons (85 and older) are projected to continue to decline an estimated 43.7 percent between 1978 and 2003 (NCHS, 1983).

Fries (1980) has argued optimistically that morbidity is being or might be "compressed" (that is, there is an upper limit of probable survival—(about 85), and the time of onset of disease and related functional impairment can be delayed and therefore cover a shorter period in the final years of life. Schneider and Brody (1983), as noted, are pessimistic. The evidence is still not clear as to whether 85-year-olds today are more or less disease-free or functional than 85-year-olds a few decades ago (Manton, 1982). Whether Fries might ultimately be right about compressing morbidity regardless of the years of survival is another matter to be resolved with evidence not currently available.

The potential for modifying aging processes and the experience of aging is not simply a conjecture. The personal and social life course of individuals and social collectivities as they age demonstrably reflects considerable social variations within and between societies (Maddox & Wiley, 1976; Riley, 1981). For example, the age at which individuals are considered old or consider themselves old, the allocation of social and economic resources by age, and the probability of and social responses to dependency vary both within and between societies at any point in time and over time. These differences clearly reflect societal preferences and values as well as individual differences. Exposure to risks that affect health and well-being with age cannot conceivably be reduced to biology.

Risky lifestyles are socially learned and reinforced. As Reynolds (1980) argues in a recent critique of sociobiology, however, social reductionism is not any more attractive or intellectually compelling than biological reductionism. The key scientific issue is the determination of the limits which human biological capacity places on the social arrangements which different societies prefer and implement. The potential for variability in arranging the life course and opportunities and expectations for the later years is demonstrably large. The biological limits of modifying aging processes and the experience of aging warrant systematic research.

To date, the principal demonstrable effects of societal experimentation have been increased life expectancy at birth and age-specific remaining years of life beyond age 65 and maintenance of a sense of well-being in the later years as the experience of the average older adult. Increasingly, experimentation has focused on the effects of modifying milieus, particularly the beneficial effects of enhancing personal autonomy, increased social support, and increased congruence between individual and organizational characteristics in special living environments (e.g., Moos, 1980; Schulz & Hanusa, 1980; Rodin, 1983; Arnetz, 1983).This research is promising, illustrating how modest social interventions can beneficially increase functional performance and perceived well-being among even very impaired older adults. The research by Rodin and by Arnetz is particularly interesting because it focuses on the beneficial effects of social interventions on endocrine functioning as well as on personal and social functioning.

The Potential for Social Intervention

If variability in human functioning among older adults is large, then human aging processes and the experience of aging not only have been but also are potentially subject to some degree of intervention and control. The key question, in my view, is not whether beneficial interventions into aging processes are possible but what processes we might wish to control that we have reason to believe are subject to some degree of control. Without making glib assumptions about the ease with which social systems can be modified in ways beneficial for human survival and well-being, current evidence indicates that learned and socially reinforced behavior and lifestyles related to health and illness and social arrangements for the allocation of essential resources which affect the selection and maintenance of unhealthy lifestyles and behavior are subject to modification. The issue is more a matter of political intent, will, ingenuity, and feasibility than a matter of theoretical possibility. Probing the individual and social limits of modifiability may be the principal challenge of gerontological research in this decade. Both the scientific and political climate for such research appear to be favorable.

We have already noted that average life expectancy at birth worldwide has increased significantly and that age-specific life expectancy in adulthood, even in the later years, has increased. Increased longevity without the complementary promise of maintaining essential functional capacity is perceived as a threat in developed societies (Lalonde, 1974; U.S. Department of Health, Education, and Welfare, 1979). In the United States, the newest cohorts of older persons surviving to age 65 are better educated, have improved access to health care, have more secure resources, and have a more secure sense of well-being than ever before. Also as noted, the "compression of morbidity" in the later years, while not clearly demonstrated, is a possibility (cf. Riley & Bond, 1983). Risk-factor modification over the entire life course demonstrably has potential benefits. In my view, the reduction of the risk of impoverishment, ignorance, and social isolation would provide major benefits to supplement the more usually noted risky lifestyle and behavioral factors (exercise, diet, stress management, drugs). And, as important as adequate medical care is during the adult and later years, what individuals can do or be helped to do through lifestyle and behavior modification is at least as important. All these changes are at least potentially implementable through public policy that addresses the allocation of social resources for employment, income maintenance, education, social integration, and social support. The potential for beneficial modification of milieus to enhance functional performance in the later years is great.

A MULTIDISCIPLINARY PERSPECTIVE
AND A RESEARCH AGENDA

Now let me return to Leonard Silk's complaint about the centrifugal tendencies of the scientific community that result in the enjoyment of dissection rather than synthesis. Both the scientists attacted to the ABMR and scientists attracted to research on aging share, to an unusual degree, an interest in the synthesis of information and a commitment to achieve a synthesis. But, as Neal Miller has cautioned, it is easier to believe that a synthesis is possible than to implement it. There is also a danger of promising more than can be delivered both in the implementation of interdisciplinary research and in the production of research that promises demonstrable benefits for older people and for an aging society. Nevertheless, serious conversation about possible interdisciplinary research ventures and the proposal of a modest research agenda relating biological and psychosocial factors in adult development do seem to be indicated currently.

My recommendations for an intersection of scientific interest among basic scientists with interests in a specific biological system (e.g., the endocrine system), scientists interested in behavioral aspects of medicine, and behavioral and social scientists interested both in social medicine and in aging are as follows (keep in mind that this agenda is illustrative, not comprehensive):

1. COMPARATIVE EPIDEMIOLOGY. Available epidemiological evidence documents fairly well the age-specific and gender-specific distribution of disease and

substantial differences within and between societies. There is considerably less evidence, however, on basic age-related biological function (normal as well as pathological) in various adult populations and subpopulations. We know even less from population studies about primary changes in a specific human organic system (e.g., the neuroendocrine system); about the factors causing primary system variability and change; about how biological functioning is related variously to disease, impairment, disability, and handicap in different adult populations; or about the modifiability of primary system changes through systematic biological or social interventions. Such information is vital as a baseline for understanding how psychogenic and sociogenic risk factors are associated with disease and biological functioning and how a change in risk factors might produce beneficial results at various points in the life course.

Attention is called here to an important study in Sweden (Svanborg, Bergstrom, & Mellstrom, 1983). This is an epidemiological study of three cohorts of 70-year-olds initially studied in 1972, 1977, and 1982 with the provision for follow-up of each at five-year intervals. The initial evidence is that each successive cohort appears to be in better health, more biologically intact. This is a remarkable observation in the period of a single decade for very old persons. The study also promises some information relevant for Fries' conjecture about the possibility of "compressing morbidity" and of maintenance of function and perhaps information on the function of specific biological systems in a social environment which is probably as benign as that observed in any society in the world. At this point I do not know the detail with which endocrine function in these Swedish research populations has been studied. The question is worth pursuing because the cohort-sequential, multidisciplinary research design used reflects the state-of-the-art in epidemiological research in aging.

Attention is called also to the research of Katz and colleagues (1983) on the relationship between age-specific years of survival and years of active survival among adults. We need very much to broaden the traditional concern of demographers to include in their analysis not only life tables but complementary tables of "active survival." The juxtapositioning of survival and active survival curves for defined older populations is essential to resolving the Fries/anti-Fries debate on the compression of morbidity.

2. STRESS, COPING, AND SOCIAL SUPPORT. There appears to be general agreement that the endocrine system is centrally involved in response to environmental stimuli. There is also agreement that individual differences exist in the perception of and endocrine responses to these stimuli, that observed differences in response almost certainly reflect differences in learned patterns of behavior and differences in social integration and related social supports, and that, with age, potentially stressful events become more probable and are coincident with probable decline of the reserve capacity of the endocrine system to adapt. The heart of the matter, it appears, is just how compromised the endocrine system normally becomes

with age and the degree to which learned coping styles and the provision of social support can ameliorate deleterious effects of stress and/or compensate for biological decrement. Answering these questions would require interdisciplinary research not commonly reported in the literature likely to be read by most research investigators with interest in aging. The best models of psychosocial stress research (House & Robbins, 1983; Pearlin et al., 1981; Wheaton, 1983) specify an appropriate range of biological, behavioral, and social variables; but rather consistently the psychosocial research currently published relies on inadequate measurement of the variables, particularly the biological variables. Similarly, research on endocrine functioning does not typically include psychosocial variables. The potential for multidisciplinary research would appear to be great. Again, both Rodin (1981) and Arnetz (1983) illustrate useful models of interdisciplinary research which includes both psychosocial and biological variables.

3. ON THE MEASUREMENT OF ENVIRONMENTS. A major impediment to interdisciplinary research on the etiology, effects, and amelioration of human stress lies in the inadequate conceptualization and measurement of what psychosocial scientists label variously as environment, context, or milieu (Maddox, 1984). In my view, the work of Moos (1974, 1980) makes a significant contribution to the conceptualization of a variety of proximate, micro-social environments (e.g., family, treatment setting, organizations). Currently, however, available procedures for indexing macro-social environments, on the one hand, and micro-social environments, on the other, are too elementary to be very useful in multidisciplinary research (Maddox, 1984). Correcting these deficits is imperative if useful interdisciplinary research on stress and coping is to occur.

CONCLUSIONS

At the theoretical level, the case for research on the interaction among major biological systems and on the interaction between biological systems and psychosocial systems appears to be increasingly strong. The methodological issues in and the appropriate research technology required for interdisciplinary research are being clarified. Implementation of collaborative research on aging which explores systematically the psychosocial correlates of biological processes such as endocrine system functioning is timely, desirable, and possible.

REFERENCES

Arnetz, B. (1983). *Psychophysiological effects of social understimulation in old age.* Stockholm: Karolinska Institute.

Binstock, R., & Shanas, E. (Eds.). (1976). *Handbook of aging and the social sciences.* New York:Van Nostrand Reinhold.

Birren, J., & Schaie, W. (Eds.). (1977). *Handbook of the psychology of aging*. New York: Van Nostrand Reinhold.

Cassel, J. (1976). The contribution of social environment to host resistence. *Am. J. of Epid. 104*, 107–123.

Finch, C. (1977). Neuroendocrine and autonomic aspects of aging. In C. Finch & L. Hayflick (Eds.), *Handbook of the biology of aging* (pp. 262–280). New York: Van Nostrand Reinhold.

Finch, C., & Hayflick, L. (Eds.). (1977). *Handbook on the biology of aging*. New York: Van Nostrand Reinhold.

Fries, J. (1980). Aging, natural death, and the compression of morbidity. *New England Journal of Medicine, 305*, 130–135.

Fuchs, V. (1983). *How we live: An economic perspective on Americans from birth to death*. Cambridge, MA: Harvard University Press.

Hine, F., Carson, R., Maddox, G., Thompson, R., & Williams, R. (1983). *Introduction to behavioral science in medicine*. New York: Springer Verlag.

House, J., & Robbins, C. (1983). Age, psychosocial stress, and health. In M. Riley, B. Hess, & K. Bond (Eds.), *Aging in society: Selected reviews of recent research* (pp. 175–198). Hillsdale, NJ: Lawrence Erlbaum Associates.

Katz, S., Branch, L. G., Branson, M. H., Papsidero, J. A., Beck, J. C., & Green, D. S. (1983). Active life expectancy. *New England Journal of Medicine. 309*, 1218–1223.

Lalonde, M. (1974). *A new perspective on the health of Canadians*. Ottawa: Department of National Health and Welfare.

Maddox, G. (1984). Modifying the social environment. In G. Knox & W. Holland (Eds.), *Oxford textbook of public health*. London: Oxford University Press.

Maddox, G., & Douglass, E. (1973). Aging and individual differences: A longitudinal analysis of social, psychological and physiological indicators. *Journal of Gerontology, 29*, 555–563.

Maddox, G., & Wiley, J. (1976). Scope, concepts and methods in the study of aging. In R. Binstock & E. Shanas (Eds.), *Handbook of aging and the social sciences* pp. 3–34. New York: Van Nostrand Reinhold.

Manton, K. G. (1982). Changing concepts of morbidity and mortality in the elderly population. *Milbank Memorial Fund Quarterly, 60*, 183–244.

McKeown, T. (1965). *Medicine in modern society* (pp. 1–39). London: Allen and Unwin.

Miller, N. E. (1981). An overview of behavioral medicine: Opportunities and dangers. In S. Weiss, A. Herd, & B. Fox (Eds.), *Perspectives on behavioral medicine* pp. 3–24. New York: Academic Press.

Moos, R. (1974). *Evaluating treatment environments*. New York: Wiley.

Moos, R. (1980). Specialized living environments for older people: A conceptual framework. Journal of Social Issues, *36*(2), 75–94.

Myers, G. (1982). The aging of populations. In R. Binstock, W. Sun Chow, & J. Schulz (Eds.), *International perspectives on aging: Population and policy challenges*. New York: United Nations Fund for Population Activities.

National Center for Health Statistics. (1983). *Changing mortality patterns, service utilization, and health care expenditures: United States, 1978–2003. Series 3, No. 23*. Washington, DC: U.S. Department of Health and Human Services.

Pearlin, L., Lieberman, M., Menaghan, E., & Mullan, T. (1981). The stress process. *Journal of Health and Social Behavior, 22*, 337–356.

Reynolds, V. (1980). *The biology of human action* (2nd ed.). San Francisco: Freeman.

Riley, M. W. (1981). Health behavior of older people. In D. Parron, F. Solomon, J. Rodin (Eds.), *Health, behavior and aging* (pp. 25–31). Washington, DC: Institute of Medicine.

Riley, M. W. (1983). Cancer and the life course. In R. Yancik (Ed.), *The prevention and treatment of cancer* (pp. 25–32). New York: Raven.

Riley, M. W., & Bond, K. (1983). Beyond ageism: Postponing the onset of disability. In M. W. Riley, B. B. Hess, & K. Bond (Eds.), *Aging in society: Selected reviews of recent research* (pp. 243–252). Hillsdale, NJ: Lawrence Erlbaum Associates.

Rodin, J. (1983). Behavioral medicine: Beneficial effects of self-control training in aging. *International Review of Applied Psychology, 33*, 153–180.

Schneider, E., & Brody, J. (1983). Aging, natural death, compression of morbidity: Another view. *New England Journal of Medicine, 399*, 854–855.

Schulz, R., & Hanusa, B. (1980). Experimental social gerontology: A social psychological perspective. *Journal of Social Issues, 36*(2), 30–46.

Siegel, J. (1981). Demographic background for international gerontology. *Journal of Gerontology, 36*, 93–102.

Svanborg, A., Bergstrom, G., & Mellstrom, D. (1982). *Epidemiological studies on social and medical conditions of the elderly.* Copenhagen: World Health Organization, Regional Office for Europe.

Syme, L., & Berkman, L. (1976). Social class, susceptibility and sickness. *American Journal of Epidemology, 104*, 1–8.

U.S. Department of Health, Education, and Welfare. (1979). *Healthy people: The Surgeon General's Report on Health Promotion and Disease Prevention.* Washington, DC: U.S. Government Printing Office.

Walker, W. (1983). Changing U.S. lifestyle and declining vascular mortality—a retrospective. *New England Journal of Medicine, 308*, 49–51.

Weiss, S., Herd, A., & Fox, B. (Eds.). (1981). *Perspectives on behavioral medicine.* New York: Academic Press.

Weksler, M. (1981). Three great systems: CNS, endocrine, and immune. In D. Parron, F. Solomon, & J. Rodin (Eds.), *Health, behavior and aging.* Washington, DC: Institute of Medicine.

Wheaton, B. (1983). Stress, personal coping, resources, and psychiatric symptoms. *Journal of Health and Social Behavior, 24*, 208–229.

Wiley, J., & Comacho, T. (1980). Lifestyle and future health: Evidence from the Alameda County study. *Preventive Medicine, 9*, 1–21.

3
AGING AND HUMAN PERFORMANCE

K. Warner Schaie
The Pennsylvania State University

Human performance is subject to vast individual differences due to genetic potential, environmental opportunities, life history, and differential societal practices in vogue at particular historical times. Thus universal principles are difficult to specify. Nevertheless, age-related changes in sensorimotor and cognitive performance present a problem in their own right as well as being precursors to other health problems. Sensorimotor and cognitive performance changes with age have been observed in three broad areas: 1) sensation and perception (e.g., vision, taste, audition); 2) psychomotor skills (e.g., coordination, muscular strength, reaction time); and 3) cognition (e.g., attention, decision-making, intelligence, learning, memory, signal detection).

The proportion of individuals in the population showing adverse changes in sensorimotor and cognitive performance tends to increase with advancing age. However, there is great variability in the extent and nature of performance change with aging. There is variability across sensory modalities and tasks in any given person at a particular age. There is also great variability in performance across different individuals at various ages and in these individuals' life-course patterns of performance. For example, my own studies of intellectual functioning show that, contrary to conventional wisdom, scarcely any individuals up to age 60, and less than half of individuals even at age 80, showed reliable decrements over a seven-year period.

Performance also differs across different societies, different historical periods, and among individuals differing in demographic characteristics (e.g., education, sex, socioeconomic status). Looking to the future, the population cohort reaching old age in 1990 will have had a reduction in the experience of childhood disease, improved nutritional history, and superior life-time health care over the current population of the elderly. They will also have a sharply increased educational background. It must consequently be expected that the old people of the 1990s will function at higher levels of cognitive performance than do their predecessors at a like age today.

Such social and temporal differences in performance suggest that biological and psychosocial factors interact to produce the observed age-related levels of performance. These multifaceted influences suggest the likelihood of a good potential that psychosocial and engineering interventions may be possible which could prevent, reverse, or compensate for age-related declines in performance. In other words, the evidence tends to support the principles announced in Matilda Riley's opening chapter.

THE NATURE OF AGE-RELATED CHANGES IN HUMAN PERFORMANCE

In full recognition of the wide ranges and sources of variability, average patterns of age-related changes in sensorimotor and cognitive skills have been described. It must be emphasized, however, that these findings refer not only to current conditions but also to current methods of testing. Many of these tests are designed for laboratory rather than real-life conditions; they omit such components as motivation or emotion; and they are appropriate for the young, for use in schools or in entry-level jobs, rather than for people in middle and later life. Moreover, all too often these tests are applied to cross-sectional samples, failing to trace age changes longitudinally in the same subjects as they grow older through time.

Sensory and Perceptual Modalities

Although there are no reliable population estimates, a number of well-controlled small sample studies exist which help to identify the major dimensions of the problem. Modalities of greatest concern (and those best studied) include vision, hearing, and perceptual masking.

vision. Beginning in the fourth decade of life, structural changes occur in the eye that lead to a lessening of light transmission and accommodation power. Thickening and yellowing of the lens reduces the amount of light reaching the retina and decreases sensitivity to the shorter wave lengths of the visible spectrum. Older persons therefore have difficulty in discriminating between blue, blue-green, and violet; reduced accommodative power affects accuracy of distance vision, sensitivity to glare, binocular depth perception, and color sensitivity. Circulatory and metabolic changes, commonly beginning with the sixth decade, lead to reduction of the size of the visual field, and decreased sensitivity to flicker and to low quantity of light. Perceptual changes with age lead to an increasing tendency to retain the initial perception of the stimulus, with consequent difficulty to reorganize that perception. Age-related decrements in visual ability have a limiting effect on the older adult's ability to use buildings, facilities, and other spatial environments, and also endanger drug compliance because of lessened color discrimination.

AUDITION. Some degree of hearing loss has been reported as early as age 32 for men and age 37 for women as a function of presbycusis. Resulting decrements affect threshold for pure tones, speech, and pitch discrimination, deficits likely to interfere with the older person's ability to communicate. High-frequency loss introduces difficulty in discriminating phonetically similar words, and increased noise level can enhance sound discrimination problems. By the time the seventies are reached, some hearing loss is virtually universal, but sex differences exist, such that men have greater loss at higher frequencies than do women and women have greater loss at lower frequencies than do men.

PERCEPTUAL MASKING. This phenomenon is the failure to perceive a visual or auditory stimulus if the sound or display is followed too quickly by a second competing stimulus. Many adults over 60 require increased intervals between successive stimuli in order to discriminate them. Longer scanning time is also required with increasing age, particularly when complex information is to be digested. It is not that the world is becoming too complex for the older person to manage; what increases in difficulty is the manner in which that person must digest the information needed to cope successfully, as discussed below.

Psychomotor Skills

Large movements made at maximum speed show substantial slowing with age due to muscular limitations. However, most movements involved in everyday tasks are not limited by muscular factors but by the speed of decisions required to guide movements and to monitor them. Changes with age in movements of the latter type are relatively small when the movements are simple and when they can be prepared in advance. Greater age changes occur when movements cannot be prepared in advance. In that case, more decision time is required, and the tendency to monitor movements is known to increase with age also. The latter may be an aspect of increased cautiousness and appears to compensate for the reduced signal strength in the sense organs and central nervous system. When older persons have sufficient time to inspect signals and to monitor their movements, they will be slower but more accurate than younger persons; when such opportunity is missing, they will be less accurate. As a consequence, in industrial work, demands for speed are often more adverse than are demands for moderately heavy physical effort by the older worker.

Cognitive Performance.

INTELLIGENCE. Age-related change in intelligence is not a uniform phenomenon, but must be differentiated by type of intellectual ability. For example, overlearned and highly practiced abilities, sometimes called "crystallized" abilities, tend to reach a peak in middle adulthood and show little decline until the mid-seventies and early eighties. Abilities involving the detection of novel relationships, sometimes called "fluid" abilities, on the contrary peak early in adulthood and show slow but steady decline from as early as the forties, particularly if measured by highly speeded tests. Overlearned abilities such as recognition vocabulary and numerical skills tend to decline only minimally in very advanced age. Those involving new learning generally begin to show consequential impairment by the late sixties.

MEMORY. Age-related difficulties in memory are also not uniform, but involve different aspects of memory function differentially. By the sixties there is demonstrably increased difficulty in encoding information, accounting for the observation that recent events are often less well remembered than are more distant ones. There is no demonstrated decline in short-term memory, but less efficient strategies appear to be used in encoding information in long-term store. In addition, there are also retrieval difficulties. These are more pronounced for free recall than for recognition, and for auditory than for visual materials. Older persons are thought to use retrieval information less effectively and to suffer from what may be termed an "information overload."

LEARNING ABILITY. There is no question that considerable learning ability is retained throughout adult life. However, the older learner is at a disadvantage when the required response time is short, and age differences in performance have been found even under self-paced conditions. The performance of many older learners is also limited by less effective encoding and organizational strategies. Older learners also suffer from response competition and other interference effects.

DECISION-MAKING AND CHOICE BEHAVIORS. When measured by currently used tests of problem-solving behavior, the major age change seems to be additional time required to reach accuracy levels shown by young adults. Slowing sensory and perceptual processes make it likely that many older people may make mistakes under test conditions by simplifying their conceptual frameworks even when this is maladaptive, or by failing to spend as much time as is required for them to obtain adequate solutions because of real or perceived pressures "to get on with it." For today's cohort of elderly there may also be a fear about risk taking engendered by the Great Depression, even though it is the older problem solver who must take increasing risks to survive well in our complex society.

Inadequacies of current testing procedures may be particularly critical in areas such as decision-making, which in many real-life situations must be based on accumulated experience or "wisdom." Efforts are now under way to design improved measures and research designs that may reflect components of cognitive performance that develop in the middle and later years. Thus, future findings may well report age-related strengths that complement, and sometimes compensate for, currently recognized age-related deficits.

AGE-RELATED CHANGES AS SYMPTOMS OF ILLNESS

Behavioral deficits frequently occur as a result of illness-related physiological changes. Among sensory disorders, for example, visual deficits common in the elderly are often a function of presbyopia as well as the early phases of treatable diseases such as glaucoma and cataracts, the incidence of which increases with advancing age. Likewise, hearing impairment most frequently is associated with presbycusis, and perceptual difficulties may be associated with mild aphasias. Sensory difficulties may be further increased due to untreated metabolic disturbances as well as to the side effects of the interaction of prescription and/or over-the-counter medications.

Among neurological disorders, perhaps the most profound behavioral changes in advanced age are associated with senile dementia of the Alzheimer type. This affliction results in progressive behavioral deterioration involving memory loss and general decomposition of behavioral competence. However, major behavioral consequences are also seen in other neurological disorders, such as Parkinsonism and multiple infarct dementia (subsequent to cerebrovascular accidents) resulting in intellectual and/or psychomotor deficits which may prevent individuals from continuing independent and productive lives.

AGE-RELATED CHANGES AS PRECURSORS
TO PHYSICAL AND MENTAL HEALTH
AND TO RELATED SOCIAL PROBLEMS

Accidents

Even modest declines in sensory and perceptual efficiency can lead to changes in accident patterns. Incidence of accidents increases with age in unfamiliar environments, as well as in those which have become more hazardous to the elderly due to poor visual and auditory conditions or where great agility and motor coordination are required. In familiar industrial settings, incidence of accidents actually decreases with age, but when accidents do occur they tend to be more serious.

Ability to Perform Social Roles

Most people are well able to maintain their job- and family-related roles into advanced age. In many individuals, there may well be improvements with aging in interpersonal competence, knowing what responses a situation requires, commitment, or ability to cope. However, the probability increases that as the late seventies and eighties are reached many persons will become unable to perform any vocational roles or to exert other than quite dependent roles when remaining in a family setting. Memory deficits, loss of adequate motor coordination, and difficulties in comprehending the complexities of the modern environment are some of the factors particularly important in creating difficulties for many of the very old to continue their lives within the community or to be adequately supportable within a family setting.

Ability to Maintain One's Health

Declines in behavioral competence associated with age may have deleterious consequences for persons' ability to engage in adequate health care. An additional common problem is loss of appetite, often associated with changes in the taste receptors, leading to poor nutrition. Memory loss and defective color vision may result in inadequate drug compliance and resulting health problems. Indeed, the lower educational level of the current cohorts of elderly may impair the ability of many persons to communicate adequately with their physicians or to participate in the planning and execution of their own health care.

CAUSAL FACTORS IN AGE-RELATED CHANGES

Although there is a massive descriptive literature on both physiological and psychological changes associated with advancing age, there is only limited information on the behavioral correlates of biological age changes, and even more sparse data on specific interactions between biological and psychosocial factors. For example, it is suspected that adverse changes in the synchrony between the autonomic nervous system and central nervous system occurring with advancing age may also adversely affect intellectual performance, particularly in job roles which require complex decision making. These complex interactions are particularly worthy of study, since a better understanding of the reciprocal relations between biological and psychosocial factors may suggest alternate modes of intervention strategies.

REVERSAL OR COMPENSATION OF COGNITIVE DECLINE

Some of the most exciting recent developments are the attempts to program systematic interventions for the prevention, reversal, or compensation of cognitive decline in older persons. This work, however, is only in the early stages of development.

Studies of my own, done in collaboration with my wife and colleague, Sherry Willis, are beginning to specify the conditions under which certain cognitive declines may be reversed. Working with elderly subjects from my earlier longitudinal studies, so that their intellectual histories are known, we have been conducting experiments to test the effects on performance of training in spatial orientation and inductive reasoning. Early results are encouraging. Substantial improvements were observed in about two-thirds of the subjects, and, most importantly, 40% of those subjects who had shown significant declines over the previous fourteen years were restored to the earlier level at which their decline had begun.

These and other recent studies suffice to demonstrate the value of intervention efforts that involve the practice of memory or learning strategies as well as the provision of incentives to increase performance. Environmental measures have also been taken to improve performance by means of changing social roles, modifying job complexity, or redesigning the physical environment.

Some of the most promising interventions involve a systematic investigation of those aspects of the physical environment which could be redesigned to lessen stress on the aging individual without impairing the quality of the environment for other population segments. Redesign efforts would compensate for both decreased sensory efficiency and lower speed of older persons. Prime candidates for such redesign include removal of safety hazards posed by inadequate illumination, glare, and noisy environments, as well as a reexamination of the adequacy of signs (e.g., easily confused colors and shapes, and spacing of information on highways to meet the needs of reduced processing speed in older persons).

Attention should also be given to the possibility of redesigning work situations to maximize performance for the older worker. For example, routine work could be redesigned to contain aspects which would tend to stimulate cognitive functioning. Although computerization might initially provide additional stress for the older worker, it is likely that attention to the characteristics of older persons in software and apparatus design may pay large dividends by reducing memory loads and compensating for losses in response speed.

Increased efforts are also needed to improve performance characteristics and to encourage increased prescription and use of prostheses designed to offset deficits in vision, hearing, and physical mobility. Of particular promise may be the introduction of relatively simple microcomputer devices serving as memory-related and other behavioral protheses.

FUTURE GOALS

For the future, goals should include recognition by health professionals that old individuals are worthwhile recipients of quality care, recognition by the educational establishment that the older learner is a prime concern of the formal and informal educational system, and recognition by business and industry of the value of the mature worker and of the need of that worker for continued on-the-job training and other obsolescence-resistant mechanisms. Equally important will be measures to get old people to recognize that most of the perceived behavioral deficits of old age can be compensated for and to encourage them to take a greater role in the management of their health and continued optimal functioning.

SUGGESTED READINGS

A. Handbooks

Birren, J. E., & Schaie, K. W. (Eds.). (1985). *Handbook of the psychology of aging* (rev. ed.). New York: Van Nostrand Reinhold.

Birren, J. E., & Sloane, R. B. (Eds.). (1980). *Handbook of mental health and aging*. Englewood Cliffs, NJ: Prentice-Hall.

Busse, E. W., & Blazer, D. G. (Eds.). (1980). *Handbook of geriatric psychiatry*. New York: Van Nostrand Reinhold.

Finch, C. E., & Hayflick, L. (1977). *Handbook of the biology of aging*. New York: Van Nostrand Reinhold.

Finch, C. E., & Schneider, E. L. (1985). *Handbook of the biology of aging* (2nd ed.). New York: Van Nostrand Reinhold.

Wolman, B. B. (Ed.). (1982). *Handbook of developmental psychology*. Englewood Cliffs, NJ: Prentice-Hall.

B. Other Edited Volumes

Brim, O. G., & Kagan, J. (Eds.). (1981). *Continuity and change in human development*. Cambridge, MA: Harvard University Press.

Knox, A. B. (Ed.). (1977). *Adult development and learning*. San Francisco: Jossey–Bass.

Obler, L. L., & Albert, M. (Eds.). (1980). *Language and communication in the elderly*. Lexington, MA: D. C. Heath.

Poon, L. W. (Ed.). (1980). *Aging in the 1980s*. Washington, DC: American Psychological Association.

Riley, M. W. (Ed.). (1979). *Aging from birth to death*. Boulder, CO: Westview Press.

Riley, M. W., Johnson, W., & Foner, A. (Eds.). (1972). *Age and society* (Vol. 3). New York: Russell Sage.

Santos, J. F., & VanderBos, G. (Eds.). (1982). *Psychology and the older adult: Challenge for training in the 1980s*. Washington, DC: American Psychological Association.

Schaie, K. W. (Ed.). (1983). *Longitudinal studies of adult psychological development*. New York: Guilford Press.

Sprott, R. L. (Ed.). (1979). *Aging and intelligence*. New York: Van Nostrand Reinhold.

Storandt, M., Siegler, I. C., & Elias, M. F. (Eds.). (1978). *The clinical psychology of aging*. New York: Plenum.

Woodruff, D. S., & Birren, J. E. (Eds.). (1983). *Aging: Scientific perspectives and social issues* (rev. ed.). Monterey, CA: Brooks/Cole.

C.   Selected Textbooks on Human Aging and Life-Span Development

Birren, J. E., Kinney, D. K., Schaie, K. W., & Woodruff, D. S. (1981). *Developmental psychology: A life-span approach*. Boston: Houghton Mifflin.

Botwinick, J. (1978). *Aging and behavior* (2nd ed.). New York: Springer.

Elias, M. F., Elias, P. K., & Elias, J. W. (1977). *Basic processes in adult developmental psychology*. St. Louis: C. V. Mosby.

Hultsch, D. F., & Deutsch, F. (1981). *Adult development and aging*. New York: McGraw-Hill.

Huyck, M. H., & Hoyer, W. J. (1982). *Adult development and aging*. Belmont, CA: Wadsworth.

Schaie, K. W., & Willis, S. L. (1986). *Adult development and aging* (rev. ed.). Boston: Little, Brown & Co.

D.   Selected Monographs and Review Chapters

Baltes, P. B., & Willis, S. L. (1981). Enhancement (plasticity) of intellectual functioning in old age: Penn State's Adult Development and Enrichment Project (ADEPT). In F. I. M. Craik & S. E. Trehub (Eds.), *Aging and cognitive processes*. New York: Plenum.

Botwinick, J., & Storandt, M. (1974). *Memory, related functions and age*. Springfield, IL: Charles C. Thomas.

Corso, J. (1977). Auditory perception and communication. In J. E. Birren & K. W. Schaie (Eds.), *Handbook of the psychology of aging*. New York: Van Nostrand Reinhold.

Fozard, J. L., Wolf, E., Bell, B., McFarland, R. A., & Podolsky, S. (1977). Visual perception and communication. In J. E. Birren & K. W. Schaie (Eds.), *Handbook of the psychology of aging*. New York: Van Nostrand Reinhold.

Horn, J. (1978). Human ability systems. In P. B. Baltes (Ed.), *Life-span developmental psychology* (Vol. 1). New York: Academic Press.

Schaie, K. W. (1979). The primary mental abilities in adulthood: An exploration in the development of psychometric intelligence. In P. B. Baltes & O. G. Brim, Jr. (Eds.), *Life-span development and behavior* (Vol. 2). New York: Academic Press.

Schaie, K. W. (1981). Psychological changes from mid-life into early old age: Implications for the maintenance of mental health. *American Journal of Orthopsychiatry, 51*, 199–218.

Schaie, K. W., & Willis, S. L. (1978). Life-span development: Implications for education. *Review of Research in Education, 6*, 120–156.

Welford, A. T. (1984). Psychomotor performance. *Annual Review of Gerontology and Geriatrics, 4*, 237–274.

Willis, S. L. (1985). Towards an educational psychology of the older adult learner: Intellectual and cognitive bases. In J. E. Birren & K. W. Schaie (Eds.), *Handbook of the psychology of aging* (2nd ed.). New York: Van Nostrand Reinhold.

4

A NOTE ON DIFFERENCES
AND CHANGES IN MEMORY
WITH AGE

David Arenberg
Gerontology Research Center
National Institute on Aging

For many years my research interest in aging has been in cognitive performance, primarily memory, learning, and problem solving. These topics in gerontology have been well reviewed recently (see Kausler, 1982), so a review of the literature will not be attempted in this chapter. It is clear that many (but not all) aspects of cognitive performance of the elderly compare unfavorably with those of young adults in cross-sectional studies; and longitudinal evidence of declines late in life has been emerging in problem solving (Arenberg, 1974, 1982a), memory (Arenberg, 1978; McCarty, Siegler, & Logue, 1982), verbal learning (Arenberg, 1983), and psychometric intelligence (see summaries in Jarvik & Bank, 1983; Schaie, 1983; Schmitz-Scherzer & Thomae, 1983; and Siegler, 1983).

This chapter focuses on one such variable—a measure of memory for geometric designs using the Benton Visual Retention Test (BVRT; Benton, 1963). Emphasis is on descriptive data; but at the end, an attempt is made to determine whether blood pressure can account for part of the declines in performance found on the BVRT late in life.

This study was (and continues to be) carried out as part of the Baltimore Longitudinal Study of Aging (BLSA; Shock et al., 1984). The BLSA is an NIH study which began in 1958 with only a few men.* Additional men were recruited until 1968 when the number of participants active in the study reached approximately 650. At that time, recruitment was reduced to a rate necessary to

---

*Women were recruited into the study beginning in 1978. Data collection began in 1984 for their second-time BVRT.

maintain an active panel of about that number of men distributed over the entire adult age range. The men are predominantly of high socioeconomic status, educated, and working in (or retired from) managerial or professional occupations. They volunteer to visit the Gerontology Research Center of the National Institute on Aging periodically for 2 1/2 days, and the study is open-ended.

Just as participants were added throughout the BLSA, new procedures were introduced. In late 1960, data collection for the BVRT was initiated. At that time, the literature on human memory/learning and aging was quite sparse and consisted entirely of cross-sectional studies, primarily of paired-associate learning. Perhaps the most comprehensive study at that time was reported by Gilbert (1941). She compared two groups (matched on vocabulary), 20–29 and 60–69 years old, on several learning and memory tasks. Substantial age differences favoring the young group were found on all measures except digit span. Those results were similar to almost all the findings in the literature in 1960. Memory for designs was one of the tasks included in the Gilbert study.

Each form of the BVRT consists of ten designs. Each design is displayed for 10 seconds, and then the subject has as much time as he needs to reproduce the design from memory. The dependent measure in all analyses reported here is the total number of errors in all ten designs.

Cross-sectional analyses for three time segments and longitudinal analyses (two points at least six years apart) for two segments were published a while ago (Arenberg, 1978). Now an additional cross-sectional and longitudinal segment can be added, and sufficient three-point longitudinal data are also available at this time. Furthermore, the three-point data (at least 12 years between first and third measures) provide an opportunity to determine whether blood pressure is related to those changes.

CROSS-SECTIONAL RESULTS

At the time the BVRT was introduced into the study, there was some cross-sectional evidence that memory for geometric designs was related to age (Graham & Kendall, 1960). Cross-sectional data from the BLSA have consistently shown declines with age.

Table 4.1 shows the cross-sectional means for several age decades for first-time performance over four periods of the study. Consistently, age differences occurred over the entire age range, but substantial age differences did not emerge until late in life.

These are age differences, not age changes. It is possible that, for some reasons other than aging, men born earlier perform more poorly—the birth-cohort confound.

TABLE 4.1
Mean BVRT Errors: Four Cross-Sectional Groups

	1960.8–1964.9		1965.0–1968.5		1968.6–1973.5		1973.6–1981.5	
	N	Mean	N	Mean	N	Mean	N	Mean
< 30	8	1.3	12	2.8	42	2.6	37	2.1
30s	67	2.6	15	2.7	61	3.1	73	2.6
40s	98	2.9	40	3.2	41	3.8	22	3.4
50s	100	3.5	37	4.5	48	4.5	8	3.8
60s	66	4.6	35	5.1	39	5.3	4	8.3
70s	55	6.3	20	6.1	50	6.6	16	5.6
> 80	8	11.8	3	12.0	12	8.3	11	9.1
Totals	402		162		293		171	

LONGITUDINAL RESULTS—TWO MEASURES

At least six years after their first-time data were collected, men who continued in the study were retested with another form of the BVRT. Table 4.2 summarizes the change data for the first three of the four groups in Table 4.1. The mean age changes were similar to the mean age differences. Little if any change resulted for the young and middle-aged groups. Only the groups in their seventies when tested initially showed substantial mean changes.

Unfortunately, longitudinal data are not problem free; they, too, can be misleading about true age changes. For example, there is the problem of attrition. Not everyone continues in the study to provide a measure of change. Typically, those who drop out are more likely to be among the poorer performers. As a result, our mean declines are probably too small.

Another possibility is that the experience of having been exposed to the test affects subsequent performance, or the two forms of the test may not be comparable. Fortunately, we can examine our data in other ways to avoid some of

TABLE 4.2
BVRT Errors: Mean Longitudinal Change

	1960.8–1964.9		1965.0–1968.5		1968.6–1973.5	
	N	Mean	N	Mean	N	Mean
<30	3	0.0	5	−0.8	31	0.5
30s	48	0.4	3	−1.7	49	0.3
40s	70	0.3	26	−0.1	33	0.5
50s	77	0.6	22	0.3	33	1.6
60s	45	0.6	17	0.7	29	1.2
> 70	25	2.8	9	2.8	25	3.8
Total	268		82		200	

these problems. By taking advantage of the fact that men have entered the study continually, we can obtain estimates of age change for a birth cohort using only first-time measures. These estimates of age change are unaffected by repeated measurement, form differences, or dropouts because they are based only on the first-time measures.

SEQUENTIAL RESULTS

We categorized the data into nine birth cohorts, each spanning eight years. The earliest was born in 1877 through 1884 and the latest in 1941 through 1948. For each birth cohort, first-time measures on the BVRT obtained from 1960 to 1976 were plotted on calendar time. The slope of the regression line is an estimate of age change. The nine birth-cohort slopes are shown in Table 4.3. It is clear that the slopes (i.e., the estimates of age change) were near zero for the latest-born cohorts and increased with progressively earlier-born cohorts. The Spearman rank-order correlation between cohort (date of birth) and estimate of age change was $-.92$.

It should be pointed out that this result could have occurred if something other than aging led to poorer scores as the study progressed. These data can also be analyzed by age group. For any single age group, any effects would be non-age effects. If these non-age effects accounted for the earliest-born cohorts showing the greatest increase in errors, then the age groups, too, would show slopes that increased as we move from the youngest to the oldest. That did not happen. As can be seen in Table 4.4, the slopes were low and the steepest slopes were not found for the oldest groups.

These results indicate that the non-age effects cannot account for the birth-cohort findings. (See Arenberg, 1982b, for a more complete discussion of this

TABLE 4.3
Birth-Cohort Slopes

Birth Cohort	N	Slope
1877–1884	16	.49
1885–1892	78	.35
1893–1900	132	.17
1901–1908	112	.35
1909–1916	167	.20
1917–1924	150	.12
1925–1932	94	.14
1933–1940	79	.04
1941–1948	61	− .03

TABLE 4.4
Age-Group Slopes

Age	N	Slope
76–83	41	.05
68–75	135	.17
60–67	108	.01
52–59	125	.18
44–51	179	.05
36–43	136	.07
28–35	116	.02
20–27	42	− .01

point.) This is further evidence that performance on this type of memory test declines substantially late in life.

LONGITUDINAL RESULTS—THREE MEASURES

Data are now available for 281 men with three measures on the BVRT. The three means for six age groups appear in Table 4.5. These ages are at first testing. By the third testing, every man was at least 12 years older. It is interesting to note that the men who were in their sixties when first tested had a small increase in errors at their second testing, but a large increase in errors at their third testing when they were mostly in their mid or late seventies. This is consistent with the large increase for the men initially tested in their seventies from their first to second testing.

It is possible that declines in health may underlie the declines in performance late in life. Analyses of performance for a subgroup of men whose health has been good throughout the study would address that possibility. One of the advantages of conducting this research as part of the BLSA is that the participants

TABLE 4.5
Mean Errors: Men with Three BVRT Measures

Initial Age	N	First	Second	Third
20s	8	2.5	1.6	2.4
30s	51	2.8	3.0	2.7
40s	93	2.7	2.8	3.2
50s	74	3.5	4.1	4.5
60s	43	5.0	5.7	8.0
70s	12	6.3	9.9	10.6
	281			

receive a thorough physical examination every visit, and their illness and med- ication history is updated.

We are currently developing a set of exclusion criteria tailored for our cog- nitive data. When we analyzed our data for this chapter, however, we had available a set of exclusion criteria for renal function tailored for a paper on creatinine clearance (Lindeman, Tobin, & Shock, 1984). Obviously, this is not the ideal "clinically clean" group for our purposes; but some portion of the men who will be excluded by the criteria specific for our purposes were excluded by the criteria used for this clean group. This group is referred to as the "healthier subgroup."

Exclusion criteria consisted of history of kidney or urinary tract disease, medications which could affect renal function, diuretics, and antihypertensive agents. Imposing these criteria resulted in the loss of about 40% in each age group. The BVRT age group means are shown for the remaining 152 men in Table 4.6. The pattern of changes is quite similar to the pattern for the entire group. Even when the analysis is restricted to healthier men, the two oldest groups showed substantial increases in mean errors over the 12 (or more) years from first to third testing. On the basis of these criteria, illness does not account for the decline in BVRT performance in this study.

BLOOD PRESSURE

One important point not yet mentioned about the change data is variability— individual differences. Within each age group, some individuals declined while others maintained their performance (or even improved). Even in the oldest groups, where substantial mean declines occurred, some individuals did not decline over 6 years or even over 12 years. The correlates and predictors of cognitive changes among the variables available in the BLSA could provide leads that help to explain why some individuals decline and others maintain their cognitive performances.

TABLE 4.6
Mean Errors: Healthier Men with Three BVRT Measures

Initial Age	N	First	Second	Third
20s	5	1.6	1.8	2.6
30s	30	2.8	2.4	2.4
40s	51	2.8	2.7	3.1
50s	35	3.8	4.1	4.8
60s	23	5.8	6.1	8.6
70s	8	5.8	7.3	9.4
	152			

One variable of particular interest is blood pressure (BP). Ever since Wilkie and Eisdorfer (1971) showed that BP affected changes in WAIS scores in the Duke longitudinal study, we were especially interested in the effects of BP on our cognitive measures.

The results can be summarized rather easily. When casual, right-arm, systolic BP was correlated with BVRT performance at the same visit, all correlations were modest but statistically significant. When the effects of age were removed statistically, however (and this was done in several ways—partial correlation, multiple correlation, within-age-group correlations), almost all of the correlations were near zero. This describes the entire group of men with three BVRT measures and also the healthier subgroup.

The results for the change data were somewhat different. For the entire group, change in systolic BP was modestly correlated with change in BVRT performance from Time 1 to Time 2, and this held even when age was partialled. But from Time 1 to Time 3, that relationship was not found. For the healthier group, no correlation was found between measures of change over either interval.

Correlations were also calculated for change in BVRT from Time 1 to Time 3 with BPs at the time of the first BVRT and with the mean of an individual's BPs at the three times of BVRT testing. Systolic BP at Time 1 was uncorrelated with change in BVRT. The correlation between mean systolic BP and change in BVRT was statistically significant, but vanished when age was partialled. Diastolic BP was not related to BVRT performance at all. The conclusion from these data is that BP is not an important factor in level of performance or change in performance on the BVRT.

A major reason for including the BVRT in the BLSA was to describe what happens to performance on a nonverbal memory task for adults over time. Although tests of memory for geometric designs, such as the BVRT, are thought to be tests of nonverbal memory, it is clear that some individuals use verbal encoding cues to help remember the designs. A cross-sectional study by Arenberg (1977) demonstrated that older men improve their performance when verbal descriptions of the salient features are heard while the designs are displayed. This finding indicates that even when verbal cues are not used spontaneously, such cues, when provided at the time of encoding, improve memory. It would be of interest to determine how subjects encode the visual information when they perform on the BVRT. Differences in encoding style may account for some of the individual differences within age groups and may be predictive of changes in performance. This was not done in the BLSA, however, for fear that such inquiry might affect encoding at a subsequent testing.

Errors on the BVRT can occur for reasons other than memory failures. Patients with some types of brain damage commit errors even when they copy the designs (see Benton, 1963). When the BVRT was first introduced into the BLSA, straight-copy performance was obtained immediately after the standard (memory) administration. Errors were quite rare under the copy condition even by elderly men who had committed many errors under the standard condition. On this basis, the errors under the standard condition in this study group are assumed to be due to memory failures.

One final point—it would be a mistake to generalize from the data presented here to other aspects of memory. It is well established that memory is not a unidimensional entity. There are several aspects of memory, and current evidence indicates that not all memory performance is age related. For example, forward digit span is little affected by age in cross-sectional studies. Generalizing those findings to similar tasks in everyday living would suggest that the old would do about as well as young adults in looking up a telephone number in the directory and holding it in memory long enough to dial that number.

Other aspects of memory are currently under investigation in both men and women in the BLSA, but second-time data collection began only recently. In the years to come, we expect to have data on age changes in several aspects of memory, and we will be able to look for correlates of those changes as well.

In conclusion, the evidence is clear that memory for geometric designs declines with age. Cross-sectional; 2-point (6-year) longitudinal; sequential; and 3-point (12-year) longitudinal analyses all indicate age declines late in life. Furthermore, the picture remains the same even when only healthier men were included in the three-point longitudinal analysis. The evidence at this time indicates that decline in this type of memory is a maturational phenomenon, and is unaffected by level or change in BP.

ACKNOWLEDGMENTS

Many experimenters administered and scored the BVRT since 1960, most recently Judy Friz, Susan Goldstein, and Barbara Hiscock. Judith Plotz programmed all computer analyses. Their contributions are gratefully acknowledged. Dr. Jordan D. Tobin provided the blood pressure data and information about the exclusion criteria. His assistance and the contributions of Diane Wysowski and the many physicians who measured blood pressure are greatly appreciated.

REFERENCES

Arenberg, D. (1974). A longitudinal study of problem solving in adults. *Journal of Gerontology, 29*, 650–658.

Arenberg, L. (1977). The effects of auditory augmentation on visual retention for young and old adults. *Journal of Gerontology, 32*, 192–195.

Arenberg, D. (1978). Differences and changes with age in the Benton Visual Retention Test. *Journal of Gerontology, 33*, 534–540.

Arenberg, D. (1982a). Changes with age in problem solving. In F. I. M. Craik & S. E. Trehub (Eds.), *Aging and cognitive processes* (pp. 221–235). New York: Plenum Press.

Arenberg, D. (1982b). Estimates of age changes on the Benton Visual Retention Test. *Journal of Gerontology, 37*, 87–90.

Arenberg, D. (1983). Memory and learning do decline late in life. In J. E. Birren, J. M. A. Munnichs, H. Thomae, & M. Marois (Eds.), *Aging: A challenge for science and social policy* (Vol. 3, pp. 312–322). New York: Oxford University Press.

Benton, A. L. (1963). *The Revised Visual Retention Test: Clinical and experimental applications* (3rd ed.). New York: Psychological Corporation.

Gilbert, J. G. (1941). Memory loss in senescence. *Journal of Abnormal and Social Psychology, 36*, 73–86.

Graham, F. K., & Kendall, B. S. (1960). Memory-for-designs test; revised general manual. *Perceptual and Motor Skills, 11*, 147–188.

Jarvik, L. F., & Bank, L. (1983). Aging twins: Longitudinal psychometric data. In K. W. Schaie (Ed.), *Longitudinal studies of adult psychological development* (pp. 40–63). New York: Guilford Press.

Kausler, D. H. (1982). *Experimental psychology and human aging.* New York: Wiley.

Lindeman, R. D., Tobin, J. D., & Shock, N. W. (1984). Association between blood pressure and the rate of decline in renal function with age. *Kidney International, 26*, 861–868.

McCarty, S. M., Siegler, I. C., & Logue, P. E. (1982). Cross-sectional and longitudinal patterns of three Wechsler Memory Scale subtests. *Journal of Gerontology, 37*, 169–175.

Schaie, K. W. (1983). The Seattle Longitudinal Study: A 21-year exploration of psychometric intelligence in adulthood. In K. W. Schaie (Ed.), *Longitudinal studies of adult psychological development* (pp. 64–135). New York: Guilford Press.

Schmitz-Scherzer, R., & Thomae, H. (1983). Constancy and change of behavior in old age: Findings from the Bonn Longitudinal Study on Aging. In K. W. Schaie (Ed.), *Longitudinal studies of adult psychological development* (pp. 191–221). New York: Guilford Press.

Shock, N. W., Andres, R., Arenberg, D., Costa, Paul T., Jr., Greulich, R. C., Lakatta, E. G., & Tobin, J. D. (1984). *Normal human aging: The Baltimore Longitudinal Study of Aging.* U.S.P.H.S. Publication No. NIH 84–2450. Washington, DC: U.S. Government Printing Office.

Siegler, I. C. (1983). Psychological aspects of the Duke Longitudinal Studies. In K. W. Schaie (Ed.), *Longitudinal studies of adult psychological development* (pp. 136–190). New York: Guilford Press.

Wilkie, F. L., & Eisdorfer, C. (1971). Intelligence and blood pressure in the aged. *Science, 172*, 959–962.

5

A MODEL SYSTEM APPROACH TO AGING AND THE NEURONAL BASES OF LEARNING AND MEMORY

Richard F. Thompson
Stanford University

Diana Woodruff-Pak
Temple University

Deficits in memory performance and cognitive functioning in aging humans are perhaps the most critical aspect of aging. In principle they are amenable to understanding at the neurobiological level. From a casual perusal of the human literature it is not at all clear that memory deficits in normal aged humans are all that great. I was greatly impressed when I read an article by Donald Hebb, a pioneering scientist in my own field of brain and learning. He wrote it in his 74th year and titled it "On Watching Myself Get Old" (Hebb, 1978). He first noticed signs of aging when he was 47. He had been reading a scientific paper and as he read the paper he decided that he really must make a note of an observation. As he turned the page he discovered just this note in his own handwriting. He had no memory of having read the paper or having made the note. He then realized that at the time he had been doing extensive research, teaching, writing, chairing a department, traveling a great deal—in fact, he was not suffering from a memory deficit; his memory system was simply overloaded. He cut back a bit on his activities and his memory returned to its "normal haphazard effectiveness."

In his 74th year, Hebb did notice changes—what he termed a slow, inevitable loss of cognitive capacity. However, these losses were not very evident to the outside world—the editor of the journal commented at the end of the article that if Hebb's faculties continue to deteriorate in the same manner as he suggests, by the end of the next decade, he will be only *twice* as lucid and as able as the rest of us!

Recent work by Fergus Craik is very relevant (Craik, 1983; Craik & Byrd, 1982). When I learned about human memory some years ago, I was taught the "structuralist" view of the human memory system, broken up into several parts:

iconic versus primary versus long-term memory systems (e.g., Atkinson & Shiffrin, 1968). I gather this view has been called into question by some workers on human memory at present, who instead emphasize depth of processing notions. Thus, Craik argues that the extent to which new information is stored in memory has to do with the depth and richness of processing of the information. In one experiment from his laboratory (Byrd, 1981), a story was read to normal aged humans and young humans. The story was given in three different versions: One was a normal version (the whole story was presented); the second was a no-theme version (the story was presented in sequence with the thematic material left out); and the third was a random collection of sentences. Normals and aged remembered material identically in the normal version; however, aged were poorer in recalling the no-theme versions and markedly poorer in recalling the random version. In other words, the more active processing required of the individual, the more difficulty the aged had.

This raises a key issue—are the memory deficits that may occur in normal aging due primarily to a loss or deterioration of the basic storage mechanisms in the brain or due instead to altered modulatory processes—what might be called depth of processing, attention, effort, whatever—a set of processes that modulate the basic storage mechanisms but are not themselves the basic storage mechanisms?

THE ANIMAL MODEL APPROACH

In order to approach this issue of age-related deficits in storage mechanisms vs modulation of storage (or of course both) at the psychobiological level, it is necessary to develop an animal model where the two alternatives can to some degree be evaluated separately. To anticipate, we feel we have succeeded in developing such an animal model: Classical conditioning of the eyelid closure response in the rabbit (see below). In brief, the hippocampus (and septohippocampal system) appears to play an important modulatory role in memory storage of this basic associative learned response but is not itself the site of memory storage. Instead, the cerebellum appears to be the locus of storage of the permanent memory traces.

The overriding problem for analysis of the neural mechanisms of learning and memory in the mammalian brain has been that of localization of memory traces. In order to analyze neuronal/synaptic mechanisms of memory storage and retrieval, it is first necessary to identify and localize the brain systems, structures and regions that are critically involved.

About eighteen years ago I decided to devote the future efforts of my laboratory to an understanding of the neuronal substrates of associative learning and memory in the mammalian brain—to continue Lashley's search for the engram. In earlier years we had focused on more elementary or nonassociative forms of behavioral plasticity—habituation and sensitization—with some degree of success (see

Thompson & Spencer, 1966; Groves & Thompson, 1970). In this work we made use of what has come to be termed the "model systems" approach to analysis of neuronal substrates of behavioral plasticity—selecting an animal preparation that robustly exhibits the form of behavioral plasticity or memory of interest and where it appears at least to some degree possible to localize and analyze cellular mechanisms underlying the memory trace (Alkon, 1979; Cohen, 1980; Ito, 1982; Kandel & Spencer, 1968; Thompson et al., 1976; Thompson, Berger, & Madden, 1983; Thompson & Spencer, 1966; Tsukahara, 1981; Woody, Yarowsky, Owens, Black-Cleworth, & Crow, 1974).

We adopted a particularly clear-cut and robust form of associative learning in the intact mammal as a model system: classical conditioning of the rabbit nictitating membrane (NM) and eyelid response to an acoustic or visual conditioned stimulus (CS) using a corneal airpuff as an unconditioned stimulus (US). Classical conditioning of the eyelid response was first done in humans (Cason, 1922; Hildgard, 1931). Hilgard was the first to study eyelid conditioning in infrahuman animals in his classical work with Marquis on dogs and monkeys (Hilgard & Marquis, 1935, 1936). He and Marquis, then both at Yale, recognized immediately that eyelid conditioning provided an excellent model system for analysis of brain substrates of memory, and they undertook a series of lesion studies with the assistance of Fulton. They used a visual CS and showed that the visual cortex was not essential for learning of the eyelid conditioned response (CR). Their results pointed to a subcortical memory trace (Marquis & Hilgard, 1937).

Classical conditioning of the rabbit NM/eyelid response (we will use "eyelid" for both components of the response; in essence they are functionally identical) has a number of advantages for analysis of brain substrates of learning and memory which have been detailed elsewhere (Thompson et al., 1976). Perhaps the greatest single advantage of this, and of classical conditioning paradigms in general, is that the effects of experimental manipulations on learning versus performance can be more easily evaluated than in instrumental procedures. This problem of learning versus performance has plagued the study of brain substrates of learning from the beginning. For example, does a brain lesion or the administration of pharmacological agents—or in the present context, the age of the animal—impair a learned behavior because it damages the memory trace or because it alters the animal's ability to respond? Or, perhaps, does it alter the animal's motivation to respond? By using Pavlovian procedures, one can estimate the effects of such manipulations on learning and performance by comparing the subject's ability to generate the CR and unconditioned response (UR) before and after making a lesion or administering a drug. If the CR is affected and the UR is unaffected, one can reasonably assume that the memory-trace system is being affected, as opposed to behavioral performance, per se. Other advantages of the rabbit eyelid preparation include the absence of alpha conditioning or sensitization, the simple and discrete phasic character of the eyelid response and its ease of measurement, and the fact that use of a corneal airpuff US permits recording of neuronal activity during delivery of the US.

One final advantage of the conditioned eyelid response is the fact that eyelid conditioning has become perhaps the most widely used paradigm for the study of basic properties of classical or Pavlovian conditioning of striated muscle responses in both humans and infrahuman subjects. It displays the same basic laws of learning in humans and other animals (Hilgard & Marquis, 1940). Consequently, it seems highly likely that neuronal mechanisms found to underlie conditioning of the eyelid response in rabbits will hold for all mammals, including humans. We view the conditioned eyelid response as an instance of the general class of conditioned striated muscle responses learned with an aversive US, and we adopt the working assumption that neuronal mechanisms underlying associative learning of the eyelid response will, in fact, be general for all aversive classical conditioning of discrete striated muscle responses.

HIPPOCAMPUS AND SEPTO-HIPPOCAMPAL SYSTEM

When we began this work some years ago we adopted the general strategy of recording neuronal unit activity in the trained animal as an initial survey and sampling method to identify putative sites of memory storage. A pattern of neuronal activity that correlates with the behavioral learned response, specifically one that precedes the behavioral response in time within trials, predicts the form of the learned response within trials and predicts the development of learning over trials, is a necessary, but of course not sufficient, requirement for identification of a storage locus. We mapped a number of brain regions and systems thought to be involved in learning and memory. The hippocampus and septo-hippocampal (ACh) system proved to be much involved in basic associative learning of the sort represented by eyelid conditioning in the rabbit (see Berger, Berry & Thompson, 1986). This provides a point of contact with current interest in the possible role of the forebrain cholinergic system in human memory and in Alzheimer's disease (Coyle, Price, & DeLong, 1983; Sitaram, Weingartner, Gillin, 1978; Hyman, Van Hoesen, Damasio, & Barnes, 1984). In rabbit eyelid conditioning the involvement of the hippocampal system is profound but modulatory in nature. Thus, neuronal unit activity in the hippocampus increases markedly within trials early in training and forms a predictive "model" of the amplitude-time course of the learned behavioral response, but only under conditions where behavioral learning occurs (see Figure 5.1, Berger, Alger, & Thompson, 1976; Berger et al., 1986; Berger & Thompson, 1978b; Thompson et al., 1980). This response is generated largely by pyramidal neurons (Berger & Thompson, 1978a; Berger, Rinaldi, Weisz, & Thompson, 1983).

Stephen Berry in our laboratory discovered an extraordinary relationship between spontaneous hippocampal field potentials (EEG) and learning of the

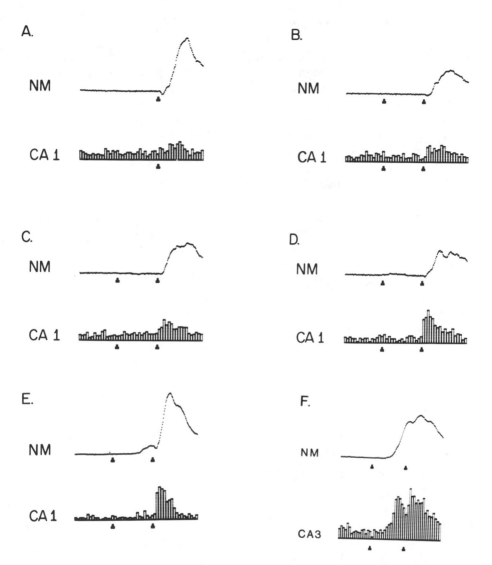

FIGURE 5.1. Simultaneously recorded eyelid (NM = nictitating membrane) closure responses (upper trace) and unit cluster recordings (lower trace) from the pyramidal cell layer of the dorsal hippocampus of the rabbit during eyelid conditioning. Left cursor is tone CS onset, right cursor is corneal airpuff US onset, trace duration 750 msec. Each pair of tracings is an 8 trial average (NM response) or cumulated unit peristimulus histogram. A, responses to US alone trials; B–E, successive 8 trial blocks over the course of initial training in an animal; F, responses from a well-trained animal. Note that there is only a small evoked increase in frequency of unit discharge in response to airpuff alone onset (A) and no evoked response to tone onset (B). Over the course of training (B–E) there is a rapid growth in unit activity in the US period that comes to model the unconditioned behavioral response. As the behavioral conditioned response begins to develop, there is a corresponding increase in hippocampal unit activity in the CS period that is correlated closely with the behavioral conditioned response (E). In the well-trained animal (F) the hippocampal unit activity forms an extraordinary neuronal unit "model" of the entire behavioral response, both conditioned and unconditioned (Berger & Thompson, unpublished observations).

eyelid response (Berry & Thompson, 1978). In brief, the degree to which the hippocampal EEG showed theta (8 Hz waves) just prior to learning was highly predictive of how fast an animal would subsequently learn the eyelid response. If the change over training in the hippocampal EEG is measured (specifically the amount of shift in the ratio of higher frequency waves to lower frequency waves), the correlation between the degree of EEG shift and the number of trials to the fifth CR is $r = -.93$ (see Figure 5.2). (The reason for the seemingly arbitrary selection of the 5th CR is given below.)

Some years ago Prokasy developed a mathematical model of eyelid conditioning (Prokasy, 1972). His model indicated that there are two phases to learning. Phase 1 begins at the time training commences and continues until the animal begins to give conditioned responses. Phase 2 extends from this point until the response is well-learned. Prokasy's model indicates that the occurrence of the 5th CR is the most reliable indicator that Phase 1 is completed and Phase 2 has begun—animals make occasional spontaneous eyelid closures that are not conditioned responses. The first anticipatory eyelid closure that occurs in the CS period (a definition of the CR) might be such a spontaneous response. By the time the 5th CR is given, the probability is low that it is a spontaneous response.

A wide range of manipulations of stimuli, training, and motivational variables influence the rate of learning of the eyelid response in animals and humans. In

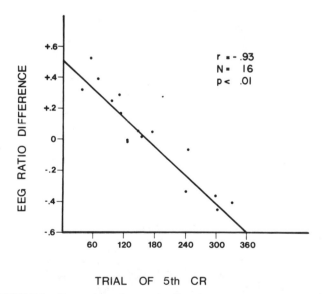

FIGURE 5.2. Scatterplot and regression line showing the relationship between the amount of change in the hippocampal EEG frequency ratio (see text) and the number of trials to the fifth conditioned response for a group of 16 paired conditioning animals. (From Thompson et al., 1980).

all cases, the effects seem to be on Phase 1—it can range from a few trials to many trials. However, once the organism has developed the neuronal substrate necessary to give CRs—once Phase 2 begins—learning rate is extremely constant. Phase 1 is the period where the necessary neuronal changes that code the memory trace are first established. It is perhaps analogous to the "processing" in Craik's terms.

In sum, Phase 1 is the period during which the specific memory trace for the CR first begins to be established; it is markedly influenced or modulated by motivational and other variables and is closely correlated in duration with changes in hippocampal EEG. The initial learning-induced increase in neuron discharges in the hippocampus occurs in the US period, begins at the beginning of training (it can be detected in group data by trial 2), and grows rapidly and markedly throught Phase 1 (see Figure 5.1).

Small lesions of the medial septum (the principle source of cholinergic projections to the hippocampus) made prior to training markedly impair learning of the eyelid response in the rabbit (Berry & Thompson, 1979). This lesion destroys the septo-hippocampal ACh system and also abolishes hippocampal theta. The lesion also greatly impairs the learning-induced increase in hippocampal unit activity. Interestingly, the impairment is in Phase 1 of learning. It takes much longer for the animals to form the initial memory trace. However, if, instead, the hippocampus itself is removed prior to training, learning proceeds normally (Solomon & Moore, 1975). An abnormally functioning hippocampus impairs learning, but the absence of a hippocampus does not. This would seem to mean that the hippocampus and septo-hippocampal system are exerting a modulatory action on the formation of the memory trace. The memory trace itself is not in the hippocampus, but the hippocampus can markedly influence the storage process. This result is somewhat parallel to the presumed role of the hippocampus in memory storage in humans (Squire, 1982).

In a striking experiment, Berger (1984) has shown that manipulations of the hippocampus can also markedly facilitate learning of the rabbit eyelid response. Animals were prepared with stimulating electrodes in the perforant path and recording electrodes in the dentate gyrus. In the experimental group, trains of electrical stimuli are given that establish long-term-potentiation (LTP) in the hippocampus. Control animals receive the same number of electrical stimuli, but at frequencies that do not yield LTP. Following this, both groups are given two-tone discrimination training of the eyelid response. The group in which hippocampal LTP had been established learned the discrimination significantly faster than the normal learning rate exhibited by the control group.

Drug effects on eyelid conditioning are also consistent with a modulatory involvement of the septo-hippocampal system in initial development of the memory trace. Scopolamine administered systemically markedly impairs learning of the standard-delay eyelid response in the rabbit (Moore, Goodell, & Solomon,

1976). A recent paper by Solomon argues strongly that this effect is due to interference with the septo-hippocampal system. If animals first have the hippocampus removed bilaterlly, administration of scopolamine does not impair learning of the eyelid response (Solomon, Vander Schaaf, & Perry, 1983). In current work, Berry has shown that scopolamine also markedly impairs the formation of the learning-induced increase in unit activity in the hippocampus of the sort shown in Figure 5.1 (Berry, personal communication).

In sum, several lines of evidence argue that the hippocampus and septo-hippocampal cholinergic system play an important role in modulating the formation of the permanent memory trace. The hippocampus is not the locus of the trace but it can modulate the rate of development and/or expression of the trace. This seems primarily to involve Prokasy's Phase 1 of learning, at least for classical conditioning of discrete adaptive behavioral responses.

CEREBELLUM: LOCUS OF THE ESSENTIAL MEMORY TRACE?

As noted above, removal of the hippocampus does not abolish the learned eyelid response nor even impair initial learning. It is not a part of the memory trace circuit essential, i.e., necessary and sufficient, for basic associative learning and memory of discrete responses. Indeed, decorticate and even decerebrate mammals can learn the conditioned eyelid response (Norman, Buchwald, & Villablanca, 1977; Oakley & Russel, 1977) and animals that are first trained and then acutely decerebrated retain the learned response (Mauk & Thompson, in press). The essential memory trace circuit is below the level of the thalamus.

In the course of mapping the brain stem and cerebellum we discovered localized regions of cerebellar cortex and a region in the lateral interpositus nucleus where neuronal activity exhibited the requisite memory trace properties—patterned changes in neuronal discharge frequency that preceded the behavioral learned response by as much as 60 msec (minimum behavioral CR onset latency approx. 100 msec), predicted the form of the learned behavioral response (but not the reflex response) and grew over the course of training, i.e., predicted the development of behavioral learning (McCormick et al., 1981; McCormick, Lavond, & Thompson, 1983; McCormick & Thompson, 1984a,b) (see Figure 3). We undertook a series of lesion studies—large lesions of lateral cerebellar cortex and nuclei, electrolytic lesions of the lateral interpositus-medial dentate nuclear region and lesions of the superior cerebellar peduncle ipsilateral to the learned response all abolished the learned response completely and permanently, had no effect on the reflex UR and did not prevent or impair learning on the contralateral side of the body (Clark, McCormick, Lavond, & Thompson, 1984; Lavond, McCormick, Clark, Holmes & Thompson, 1981; Lincoln, McCormick, & Thompson, 1982; McCormick et al. 1981, McCormick, Clark, Lavond, &

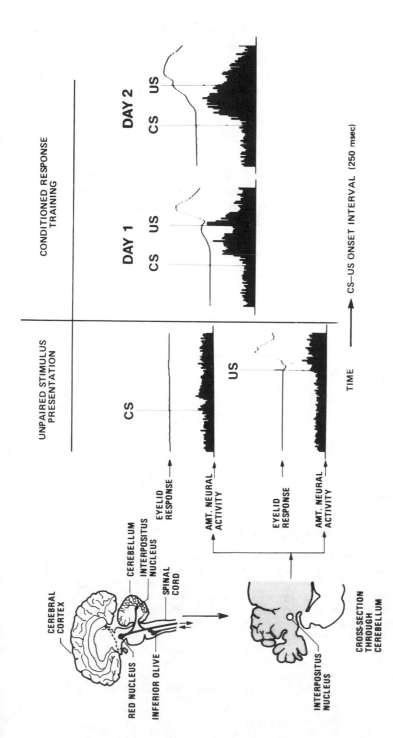

FIGURE 5.3. Histograms of unit recordings obtained from a chronic electrode implanted at the lateral border of the interpositus nucleus. The animal was first given random, unpaired presentations of the tone and airpuff (104 trials of each stimulus) and then trained with two days of paired training (117 trials each day). Each histogram is an average over the entire day of training indicated. The upper trace represents movement of the NM. The first vertical line represents the onset of the tone CS, while the second line represents the onset of the corneal airpuff US. Each histogram bar is 9 milliseconds in duration. Notice that these neurons develop a model of the conditioned but not unconditioned response during learning, and that this neuronal model precedes the learned behavioral response substantially in time (adapted from McCormick, & Thompson, 1984).

Thompson, 1982; McCormick, Guyer, & Thompson, 1982; Thompson, 1986) (see Figure 5.4). After our initial papers were published, Yeo, Glickstein and associates replicated our basic lesion result for the interpositus nucleus, using light as well as tone CSs and a periorbital shock US (we had used corneal airpuff US), thus extending the generality of the results (Yeo, Hardiman, & Glickstein, 1984).

Electrolytic or aspiration lesions of the cerebellum cause degeneration in the inferior olive—the lesion-abolition of the learned response could be due to olivary degeneration rather than cerebellar damage, per se. We made kainic acid lesions of the interpositus—a lesion as small as a cubic millimeter in the lateral anterior interpositus permanently and selectively abolished the learned response with no attendant degeneration in the inferior olive (Lavond, Hembree, & Thompson, 1985). Additional work suggests that the lesion result holds across CS modalities, skeletal response systems, species, and perhaps with instrumental contingencies as well (Donegan, Lowry, & Thompson, 1983; Polenchar, Patterson, Lavond,

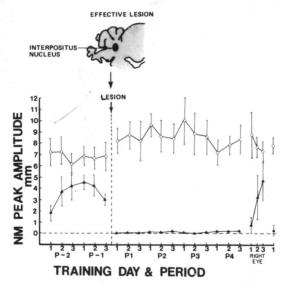

FIGURE 5.4.   Effects of ablation of left lateral cerebellum on the learned NM/eyelid response (six animals). Solid triangles, amplitude of conditioned response (CR); open diamonds, amplitude of unconditioned response (UCR). All training was to left eye (ipsilateral to lesion) except where labelled "R" (for right eye). The cerebellar lesion completely and permanently abolished the CR of the ipsilateral eye but had no effect on the UCR. P_1 and P_2 indicate initial learning on the two days prior to the lesion. $L_1 - L_4$ are four days of post-operative training to the left eye. The right eye was then trained and learned rapidly (R), thus controlling for nonspecific lesion effects. The left eye was again trained and showed no learning. Numbers on abscissa indicate 40 trial periods, except for "right eye" which are 24 trial periods (adapted from McCormick, Clark, Lavond, & Thompson, 1982).

& Thompson, 1985; Yeo et al., 1984). Electrical microstimulation of the interpositus nucleus in untrained animals elicits behavioral responses by way of the superior cerebellar peduncle, for example, eyeblink, leg-flexion, the nature of the response being determined by the locus of the electrode (McCormick & Thompson, 1984a,b) (see Figure 5.5). Collectively, these data build a case that the memory traces are afferent to the efferent fibers of the superior cerebellar peduncle, i.e., in interpositus, cerebellar cortex or systems for which the cerebellum is a mandatory efferent.

The essential efferent CR pathway appears to consist of fibers exiting from the interpositus nucleus ipsilateral to the trained side of the body in the superior cerebellar peduncle, crossing to relay in the contralateral magnocellular division of the red nucleus and crossing back to descend in the rubral pathway to act ultimately on motor neurons (Chapman, Steinmetz, & Thompson, 1985; Haley, Lavond, & Thompson, 1983; Lavond et al., 1981; Madden, Haley, Barchas, & Thompson, 1983; McCormick, Guyer, & Thompson, 1982; Rosenfield, Devydaitis, & Moore, 1985). Possible involvement of other efferent systems in control of the CR has not yet been determined, but descending systems taking origin rostral to the midbrain are not necessary for learning or retention of the CR, as noted above (see Figure 5.6).

Recent lesion and microstimulation evidence suggests that the essential US reinforcing pathway, the necessary and sufficient pathway conveying information about the US to the cerebellar memory trace circuit, is climbing fibers from the dorsal accessory olive (DAO) projecting via the inferior cerebellar peduncle (see Figure 5.6). Thus, lesions of the appropriate region of the DAO prevent acquisition and produce normal extinction of the behavioral CR with continued paired training in already trained animals (McCormick, Steinmetz, & Thompson, 1985). Electrical microstimulation of this same region elicits behavioral responses and serves as an effective US for normal learning of behavioral CRs; the exact behavioral response elicited by DAO stimulation is learned as a normal CR to a CS (Mauk, Steinmetz, & Thompson, 1986). The inferior olive-climbing fiber system also plays an important role in adaptation of the vestibulo-ocular reflex, as noted above, and in recovery from motor abnormalities induced by labyrinthine lesions (Llinas, Walton, & Hillman, 1975).

Lesion and microstimulation data suggest that the essential CS pathway includes mossy fiber projections to the cerebellum via the pontine nuclei (see Figure 5.6). Thus, sufficiently large lesions of the middle cerebellar peduncle prevent acquisition and immediately abolish retention of the eyelid CR to all modalities of CS (Solomon, Lewis, LoTurco, Steinmetz, & Thompson, 1986), whereas lesions in the pontine nuclear region can selectively abolish the eyelid CR to an acoustic CS (Steinmetz, Rosen, Chapman, Lavond, & Thompson, 1986). Electrical microstimulation of the mossy fiber system serves as a very effective CS, producing rapid learning, on average more rapid than with peripheral CSs, when paired with, e.g., a corneal airpuff US (Steinmetz, Lavond, & Thompson, 1985;

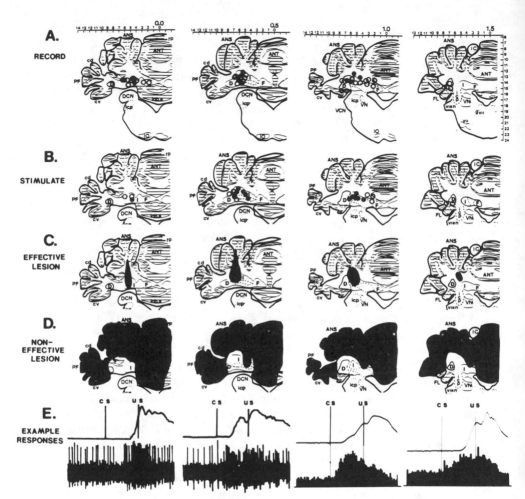

FIGURE 5.5. Spatial distribution of recording, stimulating, effective, and noneffective lesion sites within the ipsilateral cerebellum. (A) Recording sites that did (filled circles) and did not (open circles) develop neuronal "models" (E) of the learned eyeblink response. Only the recording sites that developed robust responses or no response at all are plotted. The larger numbers above each section represent millimeters anterior to lambda and the numbers to the side represent millimters below bone at lambda. (B) Sites that, when stimulated, did (filled circles) and did not (open) elicit eyeblink responses. (C) An example of a lesion of the dentate and interpositus (D-I) nuclei which permanently abolished the learned response (3). (D) Composite from three animals of cortical lesions that were not effective in abolishing the learned eyeblink response. (E) Neuronal responses of four different recording sites within the cerebellum. The first recording is an example of mulitple-unit activity from the ansiform cortex. The second recording and the two histograms on the right were obtained from the D-I nuclei. The histograms are averages of an entire session of training. The first verticle line represents the onset of the tone, and the second represents the onset of the airpuff. Each histogram bar is 9 msec wide, and the length of the entire trace is 750 msec. The top trace in each section is the movement of the NM with "up" being extension across the eyeball. Abbreviations: Ans, ansiform lobule (crus I and crus II); Ant, anterior lobule; Fl, flocculus, D, dentate nucleus; DCN, dorsal cochlear nucleus; F, fastigial nucleus; I, interpositus nucleus; IC, interior colliculus; IO, inferior olive; lob a, lobulus A (nodulus); PF, paraflocculus; VN, vestibular nuclei; CD, dorsal crus; CV, ventral crus; G VII, genu of the tract of the seventh nerve; ICP, inferior cerebellar peduncle; VII, seventh (facial) nucleus; VCN, ventral cochlear nucleus; CS, conditioned stimulus; and US, unconditioned stimulus. (From McCormick & Thompson, 1984).

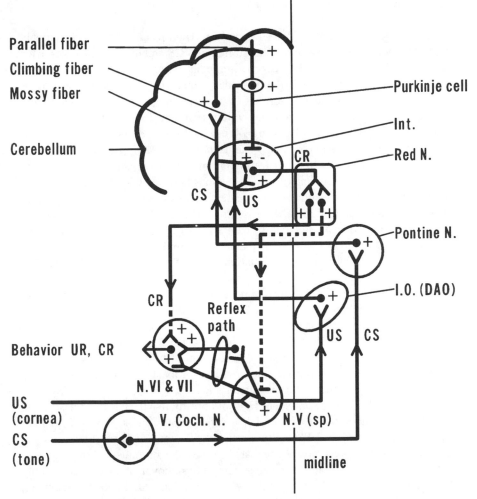

FIGURE 5.6. Simplified schematic of hypothetical memory trace circuit for discrete behavioral responses learned as adaptations to aversive events. The US (corneal airpuff) pathway seems to consist of somatosensory projections to the dorsal accessory portion of the inferior olive (DAO) and its climbing fiber projections to the cerebellum. The tone CS pathway seems to consist of auditory projections to pontine nuclei (Pontine N) and their mossy fiber projections to the cerebellum. The efferent (eyelid closure) CR pathway projects from the interpositus nucleus (Int) of the cerebellum to the red nucleus (Red N) and via the descending rubral pathway to act ultimately on motor neurons. The red nucleus may also exert inhibitory control over the transmission of somatic sensory information about the US to the inferior olive (IO), so that when a CR occurs (eyelid closes), the red nucleus dampens US activation of climbing fibers. Evidence to date is most consistent with storage of the memory traces in localized regions of cerebellar cortex and possibly interpositus nucleus as well. Pluses indicate excitatory and minuses inhibitory synaptic action. Additional abbreviations: N V (sp), spinal fifth cranial nucleus; N VI, sixth cranial nucleus; N VII, seventh cranial nucleus; V Coch N, ventral cochlear nucleus. (From Thompson, 1986).

Steinmetz, Rosen, Woodruff-Pak, Lavond, & Thompson, in press). If animals are trained with a left pontine nuclear stimulation CS and then tested for transfer to right pontine stimulation, transfer is immediate (i.e., 1 trial) if the two electrodes have similar locations in the two sides, suggesting that at least under these conditions the traces are not formed in the pontine nuclei but rather in the cerebellum, probably beyond the mossy fiber terminals (Steinmetz et al., 1986). Finally, appropriate forward pairing of mossy fiber stimulation as a CS and climbinb fiber stimulation as a US yields *normal behavioral learning* of the response elicited by climbing fiber stimulation (Steinmetz, Lavond, & Thompson, 1985). Lesion of the interpositus abolishes both the CR and the UR in this paradigm. All of these results taken together would seem to build an increasingly strong case for localization of the essential memory traces to the cerebellum, particularly in "reduced" preparation with stimulation of mossy fibers as the CS and climbing fibers as the US. In the normal animal trained with peripheral stimuli, the possibility of trace formation in brain stem structures has not yet been definitvely ruled out.

We initially suggested that the memory traces might be formed in cerebellar cortex (McCormick et al., 1981); as Eccles and others have stressed, there is a vastly greater neuronal machinery there than in the interpositus nucleus. However, we have not yet found any cerebellar cortical lesion that permanently abolishes the CR. Yeo, Hardiman, & Glickstein (1985), using rather different stimulus and training conditions (that yield less robust learning), reported that complete removal of the cortex of Larsell's lobule H VI permanently abolished the eyelid CR. Complete removal of H VI did not abolish the CR in three separate studies in our laboratory (McCormick & Thompson, 1984a,b; Woodruff-Pak, Lavond, & Thompson, 1985; Woodruff-Pak, Lavond, Logan, Steinmetz, & Thompson, 1985). Recently, we repeated exactly the stimulus and training conditions of Yeo et al., and found that complete removal of H VI causes only transient loss of the CR; all animals eventually relearned (Lavond, Steinmetz, Yokaitis, Lee, & Thompson, 1986). But these results do not rule out multiple parallel cortical sites (and interpositus as well?). Cortical lesions to date may not have removed all such sites; thus the flocculus has not been lesioned and it has recently been found that electrical microstimulation of the flocculus can elicit eyeblinks in the rabbit (Nagao, Ito, & Karachot, 1984). In general, the larger the cerebellar cortical lesion the more pronounced and prolonged is the transient loss of the CR. Further, cerebellar cortical lesions prior to training can prevent learning in some animals (McCormick, 1983). The possibility of multiple cortical sites is consistent with the organization of somatosensory projections to cerebellum (Kassel, Shambes, & Welker, 1984; Shambes, Gibson, & Welker, 1978). In current work we have compared electrical stimulation of the dorsolateral pontine nucleus (DLPN) and lateral reticular nucleus (LRN) as CSs. When paired with a peripheral US (corneal airpuff), both yield normal and rapid learning (Knowlton, Lavond, Steinmetz, & Thompson, 1985; Steinmetz, Lavond, &

Thompson, 1985). The DLPN projects almost exclusively to an intermediate region of cerebellar cortex whereas the LRN projects in significant part to the interpositus nucleus (Chan-Palay, 1977; Bloedel & Courville, 1981; Brodal, 1975). Under these conditions, a lesion limited to the general region of cerebellar cortex receiving projections from the DLPN completely and permanently abolishes the CR to the DLPN stimulation CS but not to the LRN stimulation CS (Knowlton, Beekman, Lavond, Steinmetz, & Thompson, 1986). We have thus created a situation where a relatively restricted region of cerebellar cortex is necessary for the CR, which will be most helpful for further analysis of mechanisms of memory trace formation. More generally, these results suggest that the particular region(s) of cerebellar cortex necessary for associative memory formation depend upon the patterns of mossy fiber projections to the cerebellum activated by the CS. We hypothesize that the memory traces are formed in regions of cerebellar cortex (and interpositus nucleus?) where CS activated mossy fiber projections and US activated climbing fiber projections converge.

Recordings from Purkinje cells in the eyelid conditioning paradigm are consistent with the formation of memory traces in cerebellar cortex. Prior to training, a tone CS causes a variable evoked increase in frequency of discharge of simple spikes in many Purkinje cells (Donegan, Lowry, & Thompson, 1985; Foy & Thompson, 1986). Corneal airpuff onset consistently evokes complex climbing fiber spikes in activated Purkinje cells. Following training, the majority of Purkinje cells that develop a change in frequency of simple spike discharge that correlates with the behavioral response (as opposed to being stimulus evoked) show decreases in frequency of discharge of simple spikes that precede and "predict" the form of the behavioral learned response, although increases in "predictive" discharge frequency also occur fairly frequently. In a well-trained animal, the corneal airpuff US onset almost never evokes complex climbing fiber spikes. This last is reminiscent of a recent report that activation of red nucleus can depress somatosensory activation of the inferior olive (Weiss, McCurdy, Houk, & Gibson, 1985). In a trained animal (eyelid CR), there is a marked activation of interpositus neurons that is maximal at about the time of onset of the US, which would presumably so activate neurons in the red nucleus. Thus, climbing fiber activation of Purkinje cells could function as an "error signal," i.e., when the CR fails to occur, somewhat analogously to the role hypothesized by Ito (1984) for climbing fibers in VOR adaptation.

AGING AND EYELID CONDITIONING

To sum up the work described above, we have shown that the hippocampal system plays a most important modulatory role in the rate of learning of the conditioned eyelid response but is not where the essential memory trace is stored. On the other hand, the cerebellum does appear to be the locus of the essential memory trace(s)—at least all our evidence to date points to this conclusion. The mechanisms of memory formation are operative in the cerebellum and presumably influenced by the hippocampal system (see Berger, Berry, & Thompson, 1986, for an extended discussion of this notion). Eyelid conditioning would seem a particularly apt model for study of age-related impairment in memory since it involves the formation of a new associative memory trace that is very long-term or "permanent." The major memory deficit seen in normal aged humans and in the early stages of SDAT appears to be in the formation of new long-term or permanent memories (see, e.g., Coyle et al., 1983). As described below, there is growing evidence for a systematic decrease in the rate and degree of learning and memory of the conditioned eyelid response with increasing age in both humans and other animals.

HUMAN AGING

The first investigators to report eyelid conditioning in older human subjects were Gakkel and Zinina (1953) who carried out their research in the U.S.S.R. The details of their work were described by Jerome (1959) who pointed out that the study was carried out in a home for invalids, with no young control group included. It was concluded that the process of conditioning was markedly prolonged in the aged invalids.

Braun and Geiselhart (1959) improved upon Gakkel and Zinina's design by selecting older subjects from a population residing in the community and by including comparison groups of young adults and children. There were dramatic age differences in the data. Braun and Geiselhart concluded that the main and striking result was the relative inability of the older subjects to acquire the conditioned eyeblink response.

Healthy community-residing old subjects with a mean age of 67 years were compared to young adults of a mean age of 20 in a careful eyeblink conditioning study by Kimble and Pennypacker (1963). Young subjects conditioned to a higher level than did old. Kimble and Pennypacker concluded that there is a difference between the conditionability of old and young.

We have recently collected eyelid conditioning data in the delay paradigm in 76 adults ranging in age from 18 to 83 (Woodruff-Pak & Thompson, 1986). Subjects were male and female university students and their parents, grandparents, and friends. They sat in an IAC chamber and wore safety goggles which held a minitorque potentiometer for the measurement of eyeblinks. Attached to the goggles was a tube resting 5 cm. from the right cornea which delivered a 10 psi airpuff US of medical grade oxygen. A 1 Khz tone CS of 80 dB SPL was delivered to both ears through headphones. Timing and presentation of the stimuli and recording and analysis of the responses was controlled by a microprocessor programmed in Forth and machine language.

Subjects received 12 blocks of trials consisting of one unpaired and 8 paired tone and airpuff presentations. The 500 msec CS coterminated with a 100 msec US airpuff. The US onset was 400 msec after the CS onset. Subjects were given neutral instructions designed neither to facilitate nor inhibit eyeblinks.

Results indicated that age differences in acquisition in classical conditioning of the eyelid response are large. As can be seen in Figure 5.7, subjects in the 20s condition most rapidly and to the highest level. In the decades of the 40s, 50s, and 60s and older, subjects condition progressively more slowly. They also achieve a progressively lower level of conditioning. The age differences in conditioning do not appear abruptly in the decade of the 60s and older. Rather, subjects in the 40s are already demonstrating a lower level of conditioning.

ANIMAL AGING

The animal literature on aging of the classically conditioned eyelid response shows clear parallels to the behavioral aging data on humans. Using tone CS and shock US, Powell, Buchanan, & Hernandez (1981), found that 3–5 year old rabbits (mean age of 40 months) required an average of 275 trials to the criterion of 10/10 CRs which was significantly more trials than the average of 175 trials required by young rabbits (mean age of 6 months). In a subsequent experiment, Powell et al. (1984) trained 12 young and 12 old rabbits in a similar

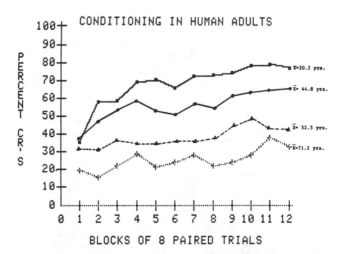

FIGURE 5.7.   Acquisition in the delay classical conditioning pradigm of 80 men and women ranging in age from 18–83 years. The age range in the youngest group was 18–26 years, and for the older groups was 40–49 years, 50–59 years, and 61–83 years. Each block in this figure represents 8 paired trials of 500 msec 80 dB SPL 1 Khz tone CS coterminating with a 100 msec 10 psi airpuff US presented 400 msec after the onset of the CS. (From Woodruff-Pak & Thompson, 1986).

paradigm but with a CS+ and a CS−. Statistically significant interactions between the age × session and age × sex effects were found. Forty-month-old rabbits showed slower acquisition, and older males learned more poorly than older females while young males out-performed young females.

While Graves and Solomon (1985) found no age differences in classical conditioning in the delay paradigm in rabbits, they did find large age differences in the trace paradigm. Eight 6 month and seven 36 to 60 month old animals were conditioned in a trace paradigm. The older group took a mean of 340 more trials to criterion than the younger group. Thus, the older rabbits took almost twice as long to acquire the conditioned response in the trace paradigm. In unpublished observations, Berry and Thompson found that five-year-old rabbits learned more slowly than young rabbits in the delay paradigm when an airpuff US was used.

With a corneal airpuff US and a 500 msec trace interval (from CS offset to US onset), Woodruff-Pak, Lavond, Logan, and Thompson (1986) found highly significant differences in conditioning between the three age groups of rabbits. These results are shown in Figure 5.8. Three-month-old rabbits attained criterion in a mean of 3.2 days (349 trials), while 30-month-old rabbits took a mean of 9.4 days (1058 trials) to criterion, and 45-month-old rabbits took a mean of 11.75 days (1392 trials) to criterion. These age differences in trials to criterion were statistically significant.

Variability between rabbits in trials to criterion also increased dramatically with age. While the youngest rabbits all attained criterion within a 4-day period, criterion performance in the 30-month-old rabbits ranged over 16 days, and it ranged over 15 days for the 45-month-old group. These results suggest that aging of conditioning capacity occurs at different rates in different rabbits. Some of the 30- and 45-month-old rabbits performed as well as the 3-month-old rabbits, while others learned much more slowly. The correlation between age and trials to criterion was .69 ($p < .01$).

Age differences in trials to criterion in the delay paradigm run in sessions immediately after overtraining in the trace paradigm were not as great as age differences in the trace paradigm. In an effort to measure retention of the

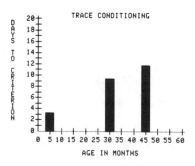

FIGURE 5.8.   Mean number of days to criterion (126 paired trials per day) in the trace classical conditioning paradigm for three age groups of rabbits of an average age of: 3 months old (N = 6), 30 months old (N = 5), and 45 months old (N = 4). (From Woodruff-Pak, Lavond, Logan, & Thompson, 1986).

conditioning task in older rabbits, five of the older rabbits (mean age = 38 months) were retested on the delay task over an interval of 2–5 months. The correlation between trials to criterion in the initial learning of trace conditioning and the trials to criterion (corrected for the time interval between training and retrainingd) on delay conditioning was .99 ($p < .01$). The correlation between acquisition of the delay paradigm and retention of the delay paradigm 2–5 months later (corrected for the time interval between training and retraining) was .95 ($p < .01$). These high correlations indicate that retention of the task is strongly related to acquisition. The longer an older rabbit took to learn the trace and the delay conditioning task, the longer it took to relearn the delay conditioning task several months later. Young animals tested for retention in the delay paradigm several months after training need little or no retraining to attain criterion on the task (Lavond & Thompson, unpublished data).

The result that 2 1/2 year old rabbits take three times as many trials to attain criterion in the trace paradigm is surprising in that 2 1/2 years is relatively young for a rabbit. The life expectancy of New Zealand white rabbits has not been empirically determined. Fox (1980) estimated that rabbit life expectancy is around 8 years on the basis of his extensive experience developing and maintaining a large aging rabbit colony. If we were to interpolate from that figure to human life expectancy, we might say that one rabbit year is roughly equivalent to one human decade. Our 2 1/2 year old rabbits which showed a deficit in conditioning in the trace paradigm are comparable in this scheme to 25-year-old humans. The oldest rabbit tested in this research was 50 months old at the beginning of the study. This rabbit took the longest to attain criterion. Fifty months old for a rabbit is middle age. Our human equivalent would be 42 years old. While we found less efficient performance in terms of total percent CR's in the delay paradigm for adults in the decade of the 40s, we found no age differences in subjects in their mid-twenties (Woodruff-Pak & Thompson, 1986). On the basis of our human data, we predict that an 8-year-old rabbit would be extremely difficult to condition and would require an extensive acquisition period. Unfortunately, obtaining a disease-free rabbit of a documented age of 8 years or older is close to impossible as aging rabbit colonies no longer exist.

Classical conditioning of the eyelid response in cats shows aging effects remarkably similar to the effects reported in rabbits and humans. Harrison and Buchwald (1983) conditioned young and old cats in a relatively difficult paradigm in which the 4 KHz tone CS + onset 1500 msec before the 50 msec shock US. CS − were loud and soft clicks presented randomly throughout the session. Ten young cats aged one to three years met the criterion of 80% CRs in a mean of 270 trials. Nine of the fifteen old cats aged 10–23 years failed to develop CRs at criterion level within 1000 trials. The six old cats who did develop criterion level CRs did so in a mean of 522 trials. Thus, old cats showed a marked deficit in a difficult classical conditioning paradigm.

AGING AND THE CEREBELLUM

Most work on aging and the brain has focussed on "higher" brain structures, primarily the hippocampus and cerebral cortex (e.g., Finch, 1985; Coyle et al, 1983; Hyman, Van Hoesen, Damasio, & Barnes, 1984; Scheibel, Lindsay, Tomiyasu & Scheibel, 1975). There are indeed many age-related changes in these structures in humans and other animals. Here we focus on the much smaller literature concerning age-related changes in the cerebellum in humans, monkeys and rats.

Ellis (1920) made a painstaking count of human cerebellar Purkinje cells and found them to decrease with age in adulthood. He found greater loss in the anterior lobe than in the hemispheres. Harms (1944) reported that in the human cerebellum up to 25% of the Purkinje cells were lost in very old patients. This result has been verified using more recently developed techniques by Hall, Miller, and Corsellis (1975). In the Hall et al. study, 90 normal cerebella were assessed in subjects ranging from childhood to over the age of 100 years. Wide individual variations were found at all ages, but a mean reduction of 2.5% of the Purkinje cells per decade were found which represents a 25% reduction over the 100 year period of life which was studied.

Assessing Purkinje cell electrophysiology in Sprague-Dawley rats, Rogers, Silver, Shoemaker, and Bloom (1980) identified a number of cell firing parameters which were affected by age. In particular, increasing numbers of abberrant, very slow-firing cells were encountered in older animals. Nandy (1981) reported a 44% decrease in the number of Purkinje cells in the left cerebellar cortex of 20-year-old rhesus monkeys as compared to 4-year-old monkeys. The number of granule cells in the same area were relatively equal in the two age groups. Purkinje neurons from old rats were significantly less sensitive to locally applied neurotransmitters than neurons from young rats (Marwaha, Hoffer, & Freedman, 1981). Marwaha et al. hypothesized that there was a senescent post-synaptic change in noradrenergic transmission in Purkinje cells. Consistent with the electrophysiological and biochemical data showing age pathology of the cerebellar Purkinje cell are the anatomical changes in old rats reported by Rogers, Zornetzer, Bloom, and Mervis (1984). In Golgi-Kopsch sections, many 26-month-old Purkinje cells appeared defoliated, with small distal dendrites and spiny branchlets being the most affected. There was a significant decrease in the mean Purkinje cell area between 6-month-old rats and 26-month-old rats. The authors suggested that the morphologic changes might be the hallmark of dying cells. In every vermis lobule examined, there was a significant senescent decrease in Purkinje neuron density. The mean number of Purkinje cells/mm of Purkinje cell layer declined from 16.6 cells/mm in young rats to 12.5 cells/mm in old rats. Related to the Purkinje cell loss was a loss in synaptic density.

Additional evidence for loss of synapses in the cerebellar cortex of the rat has been provided by Glick and Bondareff (1979). Numbers of synapses were compared in the cerebellar cortex of 12-month-old and 25-month-old rats, and the total number of axodendritic synapses was found to be 24% lower in the older rats. While there were no age differences in synapses on dendritic shafts, there was a 33% decrease in synapses involving the spines in older rats. Glick and Bondareff hypothesized that granule cells, the axons of which form the majority of synaptic contacts with dendritic spines of Purkinje cells may be preferentially impaired. The age-related loss of axo-spinous synapses may also depend upon the involvement of a specific population of postsynaptic cells (i.e., Purkinje cells), which are known to decrease with age.

Undertaking a comparative neuropathological study of aging using the brains of 47 species of vertebrates, Dayan (1971) observed that changes in the cerebellum generally resembled those seen in other parts of the brain. However, the loss of Purkinje cells was readily apparent. Indeed, Dayan concluded that there is a generalized loss of neurons in the brain "most easily detected as fall-out of Purkinje cells from the cerebellar cortex." (Dayan, 1971, p. 37).

With regard to the two major input systems in the hypothetical schematic for classical conditioning of discrete adaptive responses (see Figure 5.6), the climbing fiber input from the olivocerebellar system providing US "teaching" information, and the mossy-parallel fiber input from the sensory systems providing CS "learning" information, data from the rat suggest that aging deficits may be limited to the parallel fibers. Analysis of the excitatory projection of single climbing fiber efferents from the inferior olive making multiple synaptic contacts onto apical dendrite shafts of single Purkinje neurons revealed no apparent change in the number of climbing fiber mediated bursts or climbing fiber spikes in rats from 3–28 months of age (Rogers, Silver, Shoemaker, & Bloom, 1980). However, measures of parallel fiber conduction velocity, refractory period, threshold, and current dependent volley amplitude in rats aged 5–7 and 24–26 months indicated senescent changes in the parallel fiber system (Rogers, Zornetzer, & Bloom, 1981). From the perspective of the model, this would seem to imply that the CS input is less efficient in old organisms.

MODULATION VERSUS MECHANISM

We would now seem to be in a position to address directly the issue of whether age-related impairments in learning and memory (of eyelid conditioning) are due more to impairments in modulatory processes (hippocampal system) or mechanisms of memory storage (cerebellar system). We report here an initial study directed at this issue.

As noted earlier, young rabbits learn the conditioned eyelid response quite normally when electrical stimulation of the mossy fiber projections to the cerebellum is used as the CS. In fact, they learn it an average more rapidly than with a normal peripheral tone or light CS. Our evidence to date suggests that mossy fiber stimulation directly access the loci in the cerebellum where the memory trace is formed (see above). A mossy fiber CS bypasses the normal sensory activation of the brain, indeed it completely bypasses all sensory systems. Hence it seems likely not to activate the hippocampus. The experiment, then, is to use electrical microstimulation of the mossy fibers as a CS in older rabbits. This study also directly addresses a major issue in aging research: Are age-related learning deficits due to deterioration of sensory receptors and sensory systems or are they due to deterioration of central brain mechanisms of memory storage?

Seven rabbits ranging in age from 30 months to 44 months (mean age of 36 months) were anesthetized and implanted bilaterally with bipolar stimulating electrodes in the dorsolateral pontine nucleus or mossy fibers. Training consisted of 108 trials per day in which stimulation near the dorsolateral pontine nucleus served as the CS. The US was corneal airpuff. Rabbits were trained to a criterion of 8/9 CRs.

Results indicated that older rabbits could be trained with dorsolateral pontine stimulation as the CS, but they take many more trials to criterion than 3-month-old rabbits. The mean number of trials to learning criterion was 529.6. This is over five times as long as the mean number of trials to criterion taken by young animals. Although the range of ages of the older rabbits in this study was limited to just over one year, the correlation between trials to criterion and age (in months) was high ($r = .67$; $p < .05$).

This study demonstrates that stimulation of the dorsolateral pontine nucleus/mossy fibers yields acquisition that is five times slower in 2 1/2 year-old rabbits than in 3-month-old rabbits.

CONCLUSION

The results of this last study indicate that electrical activation of what we think is the direct input to the loci of memory trace formation in the cerebellum in eyelid conditioning results in significantly poorer acquisition in older animals, as is the case with normal peripheral tone and light CSs in older animals. This result is closely consistent with the findings of Rogers et al. (1980, 1981) that the excitatory actions of parallel fiber synapses on Purkinje cells are significantly weakened in the aged rat cerebellum, whereas climbing fiber activation is not. Since our data suggest that climbing fiber activation is the necessary and sufficient US or "teaching" input to the cerebellar memory trace system, then it may be that the "reinforcing value" of the US is not altered in the aged animal.

Hence it seems likely that age-related impairments in long-term memory storage are due in significant part to impairment in the central brain mechanisms of memory storage rather than simply to alterations in modulatory processes, at least for learning of discrete, adaptive behavioral responses learned to deal with aversive events. Similarly, this age-related learning and memory deficit cannot be blamed on decreased functional efficacy of sensory receptors and/or primary sensory systems. So we would seem to end by disagreeing with Craik, at least in that the basic mechanisms of memory storage seem to be impaired in the aged mammal.

REFERENCES

Alkon, D. L. (1979). Voltage-dependent calcium and potassium ion conductances: A contingency mechanism for an associative learning model. *Science, 205*, 810–816.

Atkinson, R. C., & Shiffrin, R. M. (1968). Human memory: A proposed system and its control processes. In K. W. Spence & J. T. Spence (Eds.), *The psychology of learning and motivation* (Vol. 2). New York: Academic Press.

Berger, T. W. (1984). Long-term potentiation of hippocampal synaptic transmission affects rate of behavioral learning. *Science, 224*, 627–630.

Berger, T. W., Alger, B. E., & Thompson, R. F. (1976). Neuronal substrate of classical conditioning in the hippocampus. *Science, 192*, 483–485.

Berger, T. W., Berry, S. D., & Thompson, R. F. (1986). Role of the hippocampus in classical conditioning of aversive and appetitive behaviors. In R. L. Isaacson & K. H. Pribram (Eds.), *The hippocampus*, (Vol. IV, pp. 203–239). New York: Plenum.

Berger, T. W., & Thompson, R. F. (1978a). Identification of pyramidal cells as the critical elements in hippocampal neuronal plasticity during learning. *Proceedings of the National Academy of Sciences, 75*, 1572–1576.

Berger, T. W., & Thompson, R. F. (1978b). Neuronal plasticity in the limbic system during classical conditioning of the rabbit nictitating membrane response. I. The hippocampus. *Brain Research, 145*, 323–346.

Berger, T. W., Rinaldi, P., Weisz, D. J., & Thompson, R. F. (1983). Single unit analysis of different hippocampal cell types during classical conditioning of the rabbit nictitating membrane response. *Journal of Neurophysiology, 59*(5), 1197–1219.

Berry, S. D. & Thompson, R. F. (1978). Prediction of learning rate from the hippocampal EEG. *Science, 200*, 1298–1300.

Berry, S. D., & Thompson, R. F. (1979). Medial septal lesions retard classical conditioning of the nictitating membrane response in rabbits. *Science, 205*, 209–211.

Bloedel, J. R. & Courville, J. (1981). Cerebellar afferent systems. In J. M. Brookhart, V. B. Mountcastle, V. B. Brooks, S. R. Geiger (Eds.), *Handbook of Physiology*, (vol. 2, pp. 735–829). Baltimore: American Physiological Society.

Braun, H. W., & Geiselhart, R. (1959). Age differences in the acquisition and extinction of the conditioned eyelid response. *Journal of Experimental Psychology, 57*, 386–388.

Brodal, P. (1975). Demonstration of a somatotopically organized projection onto the paramedian lobule and the anterior lobe from the lateral reticular nucleus. An experimental study with the horseradish peroxidase method. *Brain Research, 95*, 221–239.

Byrd, M. (1981). Age differences in memory for prose passages. Unpublished Ph.D. thesis, University of Toronto.

Cason, H. (1922). The conditioned eyelid reaction. *Journal of Experimental Psychology, 5*, 153–196.

Chan-Palay, V. (1977). *Cerebellar dentate nucleus, organization, cytology and transmitters*. Berlin: Springer-Verlag.

Chapman, P. F., Steinmetz, J. E., & Thompson, R. F. (1985). Classical conditioning of the rabbit eyeblink does not occur with stimulation of the cerebellar nuclei as the unconditioned stimulus. *Neuroscience Abstracts, 11*, 835.

Clark, G. A., McCormick, D. A., Lavond, D. G., & Thompson, R. F. (1984). Effects of lesions of cerebellar nuclei on conditioned behavioral and hippocampal neuronal responses. *Brain Research, 291*, 125–136.

Cohen, D. H. (1980). The functional neuroanatomy of a conditioned response. In R. F. Thompson, L. H. Hicks, & B. V. Shryrkov (Eds.), *Neural mechanisms of good-directed behavior and learning* (pp. 283–302). New York: Academic Press.

Coyle, J. T., Price, D. L., & DeLong, M. R. (1983). Alzheimer's disease: A disorder of central cholinergic innervation. *Science, 219*, 1184–1190.

Craik, F. I. M. (1983). Age differences in remembering. In N. Butters & L. R. Squire (Eds.), *The neuropsychology of memory*. New York: The Guilford Press.

Craik, F. I. M. & Byrd, M. (1982). Aging and cognitive deficits: The role of attentional resources. In F. I. M. Craik & S. E. Trehub (Eds.), *Aging and cognitive processes*. New York: Plenum Press.

Dayan, D. A. (1971). Comparative neuropathology of ageing: Studies on the brains of 47 species of vertebrates. *Brain, 94*, 31–42.

Donegan, N. H., Foy, M. R., & Thompson, R. F. (1985). Neuronal responses of the rabbit cerebellar cortex during performance of the classically conditioned eyelid response. *Neuroscience Abstracts, 11*, 835.

Donegan, N. H., Lowry, R. W., & Thompson, R. F. (1983). Effects of lesioning cerebellar nuclei on conditioned leg-flexion responses. *Neuroscience Abstracts, 9*, 331.

Ellis, R. S. (1920). Norms for some structural changes in the human cerebellum from birth to old age. *Journal of Comparative Neurology, 32*, 1–34.

Finch, C. E. (in press). Neural and endocrine determinants of senescence: Investigation of causality and reversibility by laboratory and clinical interventions. In H. Warner (Ed.), *Modern biological theories of aging*. New York: Raven.

Fox, R. R. (1980). The rabbit (Oryctolagus cuniculus) and research on aging. *Experimental Aging Research, 6*, 235–248.

Foy, M. R., & Thompson, R. F. (1986). Single unit analysis of Purkinje cell discharge in classically conditioned and untrained rabbits. *Neuroscience Abstracts, 12*, 518.

Gakkel, L. B., & Zinina, N. V. (1953). Changes of higher nerve function in people over 60 years of age. *Fiziolog. Zhurnal, 39*, 533–539.

Glick, R., & Bondareff, W. (1979). Loss of synapses in the cerebellar cortex of the senescent rat. *Journal of Gerontology, 34*, 818–822.

Graves, C. A. & Solomon, P. R. (1985). Age related disruption of trace but not delay classical conditioning of the rabbit's nictitating membrane response. *Behavioral Neuroscience, 99*, 88–96.

Groves, P. M., & Thompson, R. F. (1970). Habitutation: A dual-process theory. *Psychological Review, 77*, 419–450.

Haley, D. A., Lavond, D. G., & Thompson, R. F. (1983). Effects of contralateral red nuclear lesions on retention of the classically conditioned nictitating membrane/eyelid response. *Neuroscience Abstracts, 9*, 643.

Hall, T. C., Miller, K. H., & Corsellis, J. A. N. (1975). Variations in the human Purkinje cell population according to age and sex. *Neuropathology and Applied Neurobiology, 1*, 267–292.

Harms, J. W. (1944). Altern und Somatod der Zellverbandstiere. *Z. Alternsforschung, 5*, 73–126.

Harrison, J. & Buchwald, J. (1983). Eyeblink conditioning deficits in the old cat. *Neurobiology of Aging, 4*, 45–51.

Hebb, D. O. (1978). On watching myself get old. *Psychology Today, 12*(6), 15–23.

Hilgard, E. R. (1931). Conditioned eyelid reactions to a light stimulus based on the reflex wink to sound. *Psychological Monographs, 41*(184), 1–50.

Hilgard, E. R., & Marquis, D. G. (1935). Acquisition, extinction, and retention of conditioned lid responses to light in dogs. *Journal of Comparative Psychology, 19*, 29–58.

Hilgard, E. R., & Marquis, D. G. (1936). Conditioned eyelid responses in monkeys, with a comparison of dog, monkey, and man. *Psychological Monographs, 47*(212), 186–198.

Hilgard, E. R., & Marquis, D. G. (1940). *Conditioning and learning.* New York: Appleton.

Hyman, B., Van Hoesen, G. W., Damasio, A., & Barnes, C. (1984). Alzheimer's Disease: Cell specific pathology isolates the hippocampal formation. *Science, 225,* 1168–1170.

Ito, M. (1982). Cerebellar control of the vestibulo-ocular reflex: Around the flocculus hypothesis. *Annual Review of Neuroscience, 5,* 275–296.

Ito, M. (1984). *The cerebellum and neural control.* New York: Raven.

Jerome, E. A. (1959). Age and learning—Experimental studies. In J. E. Birren (Ed.), *Handbook of aging and the individual.* Chicago: University of Chicago Press.

Kandel, E. R., & Spencer, W. A. (1968). Cellular neurophysiological approaches in the study of learning. *Physiological Review, 48,* 65–134.

Kassel, J., Shambes, G. M., & Welker, W. (1984). Fractured cutaneous projections to the granule cell layer of the posterior cerebellar hemisphere of the domestic cat. *Journal of Comparative Neurology, 225,* 458–468.

Kimble, G. A., & Pennypacker, H. S. (1963). Eyelid conditioning in young and aged subjects. *Journal of Genetic Psychology, 103,* 283–289.

Knowlton, B. J., Lavond, D. G., Steinmetz, J. E., & Thompson, R. F. (1985). Eyeblink conditioning using LRN stimulation as a CS is abolished by lesions of the cerebellar nuclei. *Neuroscience Abstracts, 11,* 835.

Knowlton, B. J., Beekman, G., Lavond, D. G., Steinmetz, J. E., & Thompson, R. F. (1986). Effects of aspiration of cerebellar cortex on retention of eyeblink conditioning using stimulation of different mossy fiber sources as conditioned stimuli. *Neuroscience Abstracts, 12,* 754.

Lavond, D. G., McCormick, D. A., Clark, G. A., Holmes, D. T., & Thompson, R. F. (1981). Effects of ipsilateral rostral pontine reticular lesions on retention of classically conditioned nictitating membrane and eyelid response. *Physiological Psychology, 9*(4), 335–339.

Lavond, D. G., Hembree, T. L., & Thompson, R. F. (1985). Effect of Kainic acid lesions of the cerebellar interpositus nucleus on eyelid conditioning in the rabbit. *Brain Research, 326,* 179–182.

Lavond, D. G., Steinmetz, J. E., Yokaitis, M. H., Lee, J., & Thompson, R. F. (1986). Retention of classical conditioning after removal of cerebellar cortex. *Neuroscience Abstracts, 12,* 753.

Lincoln, J. S., McCormick, D. A., & Thompson, R. F. (1982). Ipsilateral cerebellar lesions prevent learning of the classically conditioned nictitating membrane/eyelid response. *Brain Research, 242,* 190–193.

Llinas, R., Walton, K., & Hillman, D. E. (1975). Inferior olive: its role in motor learning. *Science, 190,* 1230–1231.

Madden, J. IV, Haley, D. A., Barchas, J. D., & Thompson, R. F. (1983). Microfusion of picrotóoxin into the caudal red nucleus selectively abolishes the classically conditioned nictitating membrane/eyelid response in the rabbit. *Neuroscience Abstracts, 9,* 830. (1983).

Marquis, D. G. & Hilgard, E. R. (1937). Conditioned responses to light in monkeys after removal of the occipital lobes. *Brain, 60,* 1–12.

Marwaha, J., Hoffer, B. J., & Freedman, R. (1981). Changes in noradrenergic neurotransmission in rat cerebellum during aging. *Neurobiology of Aging, 2,* 95–98.

Mauk, M. D., Steinmetz, J. E., & Thompson, R. F. (1986). Classical conditioning using stimulation of the inferior olive as the unconditioned stimulus. *Proceedings of the National Academy of Sciences,* USA, *83,* 5349–5353.

Mauk, M. D., & Thompson, R. F. (in press). Retention of classically conditioned eyelid responses following acute decerebration. *Brain Research.*

McCormick, D. A. (1983). *Cerebellum: Essential involvement in a simple learned response.* Unpublished doctoral dissertation, Stanford University.

McCormick, D. A., & Thompson, R. F. (1984a). Cerebellum: Essential involvement in the classically conditioned eyelid response. *Science, 223,* 296–299.

McCormick, D. A., & Thompson, R. F. (1984b). Neuronal responses of the rabbit cerebellum during acquisition and performance of a classically conditioned nictitating membrane-eyelid response. *Journal of Neuroscience, 4*(11), 2811–2822.

McCormick, D. A., Lavond, D. G., Clark, G. A., Kettner, R. E., Rising, C. E., & Thompson, R. F. (1981). The engram found? Role of the cerebellum in classical conditioning of nictitating membrane and eyelid responses. *Bulletin of the Psychological Society, 18*(3), 103–105.

McCormick, D. A., Clark, G. A., Lavond, D. G., & Thompson, R. F. (1982). Initial localization of the memory trace for a basic form of learning. *Proceedings of the National Academy of Sciences, 79*(8), 2731–2742.

McCormick, D. A., Guyer, P. E., & Thompson, R. F. (1982). Superior cerebellar peduncle selectively abolish the ipsilateral calssically conditioned nictitating membrane/eyelid response of the rabbit. *Brain Research, 244*, 347–350.

McCormick, D. A., Lavond, D. G., & Thompson, R. F. (1983). Neuronal responses of the rabbit brainstem during performance of the classically conditioned nictitating membrane (NM) eyelid response. *Brain Research, 271*, 73–88.

McCormick, D. A., Steinmetz, J. E., & Thompson, R. F. (1985). Lesions of the inferior olivary complex cause extinction of the classically conditioned eyeblink response. *Brain Research, 359*, 120–130.

Moore, J. W., Goodell, N. A., & Solomon, P. R. (1976). Central cholinergic blockage by scopolamine and habituation, classical conditioning, and latent inhibition of the rabbit's nictitating membrane response. *Physiological Psychology, 4*, 395–399.

Nagao, S., Ito, M., & Karachot, L. (1984). Sites in the rabbit flocculus specifically related to eye blinking and neck muscle contraction. *Neuroscience Research, 1*, 149–152.

Nandy, K. (1981). Morphological changes in the cerebellar cortex of aging *Macaca nemestrina*. *Neurobiology of Aging, 2*, 61–64.

Norman, R. J., Buchwald, J. S., & Villablanca, J. R. (1977). Classical conditioning with auditory discrimination of the eyeblink in decerebrate cats. *Science, 196*, 551–553.

Oakley, D. A., & Russel, I. S. (1977). Subcortical storage of Pavlovian conditioning in the rabbit. *Physiology and Behavior, 18*, 931–937.

Polenchar, B. E., Patterson, M. M., Lavond, D. G., & Thompson, R. F. (1985). Cerebellar lesions abolish an avoidance response in rabbit. *Behavioral and Neural Biology, 44*, 221–227.

Powell, D. A., Buchanan, S. L., & Hernandez, L. L. (1981). Age related changes in classical (Pavlovian) conditioning in the New Zealand albino rabbit. *Experimental Aging Research, 7*, 453–465.

Powell, D. A., Buchanan, S. L., & Hernandez, L. L. (1984). Age-related changes in Pavlovian conditioning: Central nervous system correlates. *Physiology and Behavior, 32*, 609–616.

Prokasy, W. F. (1972). In A. H. Black & W. F. Prokasy (Eds.), *Classical conditioning II: Current theory and research*. New York: Appleton.

Rogers, J., Silver, M. A., Shoemaker, W. J., & Bloom, F. E. (1980). Cerebellar Purkinje cell electrophysiology and correlative anatomy. *Neurobiology of Aging, 1*, 3–11.

Rogers, J., Zornetzer, S. F., & Bloom, F. E. (1981). Senescent pathology of cerebellum: Purkinje neurons and their parallel fiber afferents. *Neurobiology of Aging, 2*, 15–25.

Rogers, J., Zornetzer, S. F., Bloom, F. E., & Mervis, R. E. (1984). Senescent microstructural changes in rat cerebellum. *Brain Research, 292*, 23–32.

Rosenfield, M. E., Devydaitis, A., & Moore, J. W. (1985). *Brachium conjunctivum* and rubrobulbar tract: Brainstem projections of red nucleus essential for the conditioned nictitating membrane response. *Physiology and Behavior, 34*, 751–759.

Scheibel, M. E., Lindsay, R. D., Tomiyasu, U., & Scheibel, A. B. (1975). Progressive dendritic jhanges in aging human cortex. *Experimental Neurology, 47*, 392–403.

Shambes, G. M., Gibson, J. M., & Welker, W. (1978). Fractured somatotopy in granule cell tactile areas of rat cerebellar hemispheres revealed by micromapping. *Brain, Behavior and Evolution, 15*, 94–140.

Sitaram, N., Weingartner, H., & Gillin, J. C. (1978). Human serial learning: Enhancement with arecoline and choline, and impairment with scopolamine. *Science, 201*, 274–276.

Solomon, P. R., & Moore, J. W. (1975). Latent inhibition and stimulus generalization of the classically conditioned nictitating membrane response in rabbits (Oryctolagus cuniculus) following dorsal hippocampal ablations. *Journal of Comparative Physiological Psychology 89*, 1192–1203.

Solomon, P. R., Solomon, S. D., Vander Schaaf, E., & Perry, H. E. (1983). Altered activity in the hippocampus is more detrimental to classical conditioning than removing the structure. *Science, 220*, 329–333.

Solomon, P. R., Lewis, J. L., LoTurco, J. J., Steinmetz, J. E., & Thompson, R. F. (1986). The role of the middle cerebellar peduncle in acquisition and retention of the rabbit's classically conditioned nictitating membrane response. *Bulletin of the Psychonomic Society, 24*, 75–78.

Squire, L. R. (1982). The neuropsychology of human memory. *Annual Review of Neuroscience, 5*, 241.

Steinmetz, J. E., Lavond, D. G., & Thompson, R. F. (1985). Classical conditioning of the rabbit eyelid response with mossy fiber stimulation as the conditioned stimulus. *Bulletin of the Psychonomic Society, 23*, 245–248.

Steinmetz, J. E., Lavond, D. G., & Thompson, R. F. (1985). Classical conditioning of skeletal muscle responses with mossy fiber stimulation CS and climbing fiber stimulation US. *Neuroscience Abstracts, 11*, 982

Steinmetz, J. E., Rosen, D. J., Chapman, P. R., Lavond, D. G., & Thompson, R. F. (1986). Classical conditioning of the rabbit eyelid response with a mossy fiber stimulation CS. I. Pontine nuclei and middle cerebellar peduncle stimulation. *Behavioral Neuroscience, 100*, 871–880.

Steinmetz, J. E., Rosen, D. J., Woodruff-Pak, D. S., Lavond, D. G., & Thompson, R. F. (in press). Rapid transfer of training occurs when direct mossy fiber stimulation is used as a conditioned stimulus for classical eyelid conditioning. *Neuroscience Research*.

Thompson, R. F. (1986). The neurobiology of learning and memory. *Science, 233*, 941–947.

Thompson, R. F., Berger, T. W., & Madden, J. IV (1983). Cellular processes of learning and memory in the mammalian CNS. *Annual Review of Neuroscience, 6*, 447–491.

Thompson, R. F., Berger, T. W., Cegavske, C. F., Patterson, M. M., Roemer, R. A., Teyler, T. J., & Young, R. A. (1976). A search for the engram. *American Psychologist, 31*, 209–227.

Thompson, R. F., Berger, T. W., Berry, S. D., Hoehler, F. K., Kettner, R. E., & Weisz, D. J. (1980). Hippocampal substrate of classical conditioning. *Physiological Psychology, 8*, 262–279.

Thompson, R. F., & Spencer, W. A. (1966). Habituation: A model phenomenon for the study of neuronal substrates of behavior. *Psychological Review, 173*, 16–43.

Tsukahara, N. (1981). Snyaptic plasticity in the mammalian central nervous system. *Annual Review of Neuroscience, 4*, 351–379.

Weiss, C., McCurdy, M. L., Houk, J. C., & Gibson, A. R. (1985). Anatomy and physiology of dorsal column afferents to forelimb dorsal accessory olive. *Neuroscience Abstracts, 11*, 182.

Woodruff-Pak, D. S., Lavond, D. G., & Thompson, R. F. (1985). Trace conditioning: Abolished by cerebellar nuclear lesions but not lateral cerebellar cortex aspirations. *Brain Research, 348*, 249–260.

Woodruff-Pak, D. S., Lavond, D. G., Logan, C. G., Steinmetz, J. E., & Thompson, R. F. (1985). The continuing search for a role of the cerebellar cortex in eyelid conditioning. *Neuroscience Abstracts, 11*, 333.

Woodruff-Pak, D. S., & Thompson, R. F. (in press). Neural correlates of classical conditioning across the life span. In P. B. Baltes, D. M. Featherman, R. M. Learner (Eds.), *Life-span development and behavior*. Hillsdale, NJ: Erlbaum.

Woodruff-Pak, D. S., Lavond, D. G., Logan, C. G., & Thompson, R. F. (1986). Classical conditioning of rabbits 2-1/2 years old using mossy fiber stimulation as a CS. *Neuroscience Abstracts, 12*, 1315.

Woody, C. D., Yarowsky, P., Owens, J., Black-Cleworth, P., & Crow, T. (1974). Effects of lesions of coronal motor areas on acquisition of conditioned eye blink in the cat. *Journal of Neurophysiology, 37*, 385–394.

Yeo, C. H., Hardiman, M. J., & Glickstein, M. (1984). Discrete lesions of the cerebellar cortex abolish the classically conditioned nictitating membrane response of the rabbit. *Behavioral Brain Research, 13*, 261–266.

Yeo, C. H., Hardiman, M. J., & Glickstein, M. (1985). Classical conditioning of the nictitating membrane response of the rabbit: II. Lesions of the cerebellar cortex. *Experimental Brain Research, 60,* 99–113.

6

ENVIRONMENTAL INFLUENCES ON THE BRAIN DURING AGING

Caleb E. Finch
*Department of Biological Sciences
and the Andrus Gerontology Center
University of Southern California*

INTRODUCTION

This brief essay will outline some of the modes by which the environment of the mamalian brain can influence brain functions over the life course and will attempt to identify major gaps in information. The commanding role of the nervous system in regulating the function of the body has been recognized for a century and a half. But it is only recently that attention has been paid to the alterations with aging of the nervous system and the neuroendocrine and other regulatory systems. (For a review of the neuroendocrine system, see Finch and Landfield, 1985.) The interactions of the brain with the environment—both physiological and social—are still poorly understood and include recursive circuits that feed back on many levels of the nervous system. For example, adverse social conditions may be transduced first as sensory information with subsequent alterations of the sympathoadrenal axis. Similarly, stress can influence sleep patterns, which may further influence adrenal steroids or nutrient flow, which, then, can reflect back on the brain. Such considerations are familiar from decades of studies on psychosomatic and somatopsychologic disorders, but may have special significance to the degenerative changes in the brain during aging because of a newly recognized category of phenomena: Steroids under some conditions cause degeneration of specific brain cells. Such effects may be irreversible and constitute a type of steroidal memory that appears to interact with aging processes. Before describing these phenomena, I will first sketch out some issues about the extent of intrinsic aging changes that may occur in nervous tissues.

INTRINSIC AGING CHANGES

In view of the generic property of nervous systems to respond to their environments, the question arises about aging processes which are independent of the environment. An age-correlated process which could be considered an intrinsic aging mechanism is the increase of D-aspartic acid in human white matter (Man, Sandhouse, Burg, & Fisher, 1983). Many studies show the spontaneous racemization of L-amino acids at body temperature which occurs on a random basis and is thermodynamically driven. Myelin, tooth enamel, lens crystalins, and other proteins which are slowly or never replaced, manifest an accumulation of D-amino acids as a linear function of time during the human life span (Masters, Bada, & Zigler, 1975; Masters-Helfman & Bada, 1975). The accumulation of D-amino acids in lens proteins may be a factor in cataracts, but there is no present correlate of dysfunction with accumulated D-amino acids in myelin.

A long-standing candidate for an intrinsic cell aging process is the accumulation of intracellular aging pigments (lipofuscins), which are accrued as a linear function of time (age). The rate of accumulation appears to vary widely with neuronal cell type (Toth, 1968) and so far has no clear functional correlate. For example, the neurons of the inferior olive, which are part of the vestibulary system, often have such large intracellular pigment depots that the cell nucleus is pushed out of its normal position; yet, there is no loss of these neurons even by the tenth decade (Monagle & Brody, 1974). Thus, age pigment accumulation may be an example of an intrinsic cell aging process that is correlated with the cell's cumulative metabolic work, but so far lacks any clear correlate of dysfunction. The discovery that neuronal pigments are rapidly induced in hippocampal neurons of young rats by the protease inhibitor, leupeptin (Ivy, Schotter, Baudry, & Lynch, 1983), gives a new experimental approach to this long-standing question.

A question of potential importance to aging concerns the possibility of a use-related exhaustion or depletion of brain cell activities in age-related brain dysfunctions. The question of intrinsic aging in brain cells can also be viewed in the context of a speculation about the nature of aging processes, articulated by T. H. Huxley (1896) ". . . the matter of life is a veritable 'peu de chagrin,' and for every vital act, it is somewhat the smaller." That is, cells might progressively deplete some putative potentials through normal metabolic functioning, which during the course of aging (time) would lead to exhaustion and senescence. This idea was extended by the calculations of Rubner (1908) and others, that the total number of heartbeats and caloric output during the life span was roughly similar in short- and long-lived mammals, and that some physiological rates of aging were scaled inversely with the life span. However, there are serious reservations about calculations of total energy expenditure as a limiting factor in life span (Yates, in press; Lindsted & Calder, 1981; Sacher & Duffy, 1979); moreover, a long list of cell activities shows no evidence of dysfunction during aging (Finch,

1976). The discovery that normal (diploid) skin or lung fibroblasts from humans had a limited potential for replication in standard culture conditions (Hayflick & Moorehead, 1961) gave further credence to the concept of intrinsic cell aging. These *in vitro* aging phenomena have been extended to other cell types (e.g., Hornsby & Gill, 1978; Lipman & Muggleton-Harris, 1982). A case of particular interest is the capacity of bovine adrenocortical cells to produce steroids: The steroidogenic responses to ACTH did not decline during serial passage in vitro, although the stimulation of cAMP production declined strikingly during the loss of proliferative capacity (Hornsby & Gill, 1978). The contributions of such phenomena to the age-correlated declines of steroid production or of neuroscretions *in vivo* remain to be established. On the other hand, there is no evidence that all dividing cells have such a limitation, as may be represented by the continued mitotic ability of some mucosal cell types up to old age (Lesher, Fry, & Kohn, 1961; Lesher, 1966). For further discussion, see Finch (1976) and Harrison (1985).

It should be stressed that the loss of cell replication by diploid cells does not mean that cell senescence or death immediately follows. Thus, neurons in the mammalian brain cease dividing soon after birth, yet many do not show degenerative changes for decades. Moreover, nondividing, "senescent" fibroblast cultures can survive for many months if the medium is changed (Bell et al., 1978), as can the ability of these "senescent" fibroblasts to support viral infections (e.g., Holland, Korne, & Doyle, 1973).

An important question is, are permanently non-dividing cells different from the above examples of cells with limited proliferation? There are few cases for discussion. First, the myocardium (largely postmitotic) can hypertrophy extensively in older humans (Van Peenen & Gerstl, 1962) and laboratory rodents (Hugin & Verzar, 1956; Florini, Saito, & Manowitz, 1973); the rate of myocardial hypertrophy may become slower with aging, however (Florini et al., 1973).

Another case is the ability of the hypothalamus and anterior pituitary to maintain a high output of gonadotropins for most of the life span after ovariectomy of young rats (Blake, Elias, & Huffman, 1983) or mice (Gee, Flurkey, & Finch, 1983) or after castration in human eunuchs (Hamilton, Catchpole, & Hawke, 1945). The mechanisms of this 20–50 times supranormal production of gonadotropins after removal of gonads appear to involve increased output of the hypothalamic neuropeptide, GnRH (gonadotropin-releasing hormone), as well as increased basal output by the pituitary (Leipheimer & Gallo, 1983). A similar increase of gonadotropins is characteristic of postmenopausal women; some studies show that the hypersecretion of gonadotropins continues for 30 or more years (Scaglia et al., 1976). These examples suggest that the hypothalamic neurons which produce GnRH do not deteriorate from the stress of prolonged hypersecretion. For example, tenfold more gonadotropins are secreted during long-term castration in mice than are normally produced during the reproductive life span (Gee et al., 1983). Moreover, there is evidence that aging does not reduce the number of GnRH-producing neurons, at least in mice during female reproductive senescence (Hoffman & Finch, 1986).

Another approach was used in the rarely cited study of Duncan and Jarvis (1943), who induced a peripheral nerve to regenerate many times. A peripheral, 2–3 mm segment of the facial nerve in cats was excised or damaged; regeneration was documented historically and by recovery of eyelid closure in response to a puff of air. Remarkably, the facial nerve regenerated up to nine times without evident histologic deterioration of the cell bodies.

A compensatory hyperactivity results from experimental damage to several neuronal populations that, in another context, are damaged in age-related neurologic diseases. Damage to the terminals of the noradrenergic neurons projecting from the locus ceruleus in young rats causes a compensatory increase of dopamine-(beta)-hydroxylase in the cell bodies (Acheson & Zigmond, 1981). Similarly, lesions of the cholinergic cell bodies in the nucleus basalis of Meynert lead to transient deficits, but with eventual complete recovery of high-affinity choline uptake (Pedata, LoConte, Sorbi, Marconcini-Pepeu, & Pepeu, 1982) and choline acetyltransferase (Wenk & Olton, 1984; Pasinetti & Finch, in prep) in the affected cortex.

In view of these compensatory responses, it was therefore striking that morphologic studies of Parkinson's and Alzheimer's brains showed a 20–35% *decrease* in nucleolar volume in the substantia nigra (Mann & Yates, 1983) and nucleus basalis of Meynert (Mann & Yates, 1982), respectively, as compared to age-matched controls with normal numbers of these neurons. A decreased nucleolar volume is *opposite* to that expected from compensatory hyperactivity of the remaining neurons, since nucleolar volume is strongly correlated with cell-body RNA content and biosynthetic activities in neurons (Watson, 1968; Edstrom & Eichner, 1958); the nucleolus is the site of ribosomal RNA synthesis and hence reflects major modulations in protein synthesis.

The smaller nucleolus of the remaining neurons in Parkinsonism and Alzheimer's suggests a new, experimentally testable hypothesis, that sustained compensatory hyperactivity eventually causes functional exhaustion in some neuronal types. The onset of symptoms thus might ensue long after the initial neuronal loss or damage, as a consequence of exhaustion from sustained hyperactivity. Such long-delayed manifestations of neuronal damage have been postulated to account for the gap of decades or more between the viral encephalitis epidemic of the 1920s and the onset of Parkinsonism (Poskanzer & Schwab, 1961). Another example of delayed expression of lesions until late in life is provided by the reemergence of sensorimotor impairments in old rats which were given lesions of the medial forebrain bundle when young; initially, the rats had recovered normal motor functions, which were retained for about 12 minutes (Schallert, 1983). Such phenomena can be viewed accoding to models in which initial lesions are subthreshold until summated with normal or accelerated aging changes (Finch, 1980; see Figure 6.1).

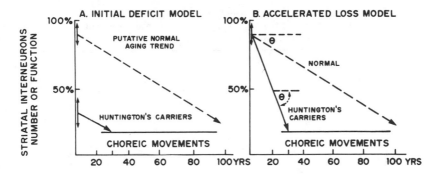

FIGURE 6.1. Two mechanisms for the age-related incidence of Huntington's chorea. The onset of choreic movements is assumed to result when deficits of striatal neurons (either number or function) reach some critical threshold (solid horizontal lines). The onset is hypothesized to occur when the Huntingtonian lesion summates with normal age-related trends for progressive striatal cell loss or functional impairment. In the initial deficit mechanism (A), the rate of striatal impairment is the same as in normal aging; the threshold for chorea is reached when the congenital deficits, which were initially insufficient to cause neurological abnormalities, are summated to threshold with the normal aging trend. In the accelerated loss model (above), the normal rate of impairment is greatly accelerated. No information is available about the time course of striatal neuron loss in Huntington's chorea (Finch, 1980). Similar models apply to Parkinsonism and Alzheimer's disease.

STEROID-INDUCED BRAIN DAMAGE IN RODENTS AND SHEEP: A POTENTIAL TRANSDUCER OF PSYCHOSOCIAL INFLUENCES ON THE AGING PROCESS

A new phenomenon was recently recognized, in which steroids appear to cause irreversible changes in the adult brain of rodents and sheep. Exposure of adult laboratory rodents to sustained, physiological elevations of some steroids for 3–6 months can cause long-lasting alterations in neuroendocrine function, with evidence of neuronal damage in the arcuate nucleus of the hypothalamus by estradiol (Brawer & Sonnenschein, 1975; Casanueva et al., 1982; Sarkar, Gottschall, & Meites, 1982) and in the hippocampus by corticosterone (Landfield, Lindsey, & Lynch, 1978a; Landfield, Waymire, & Lynch, 1978b). Most recently, intriguing but limited evidence suggests that hippocampal pyamidal neurons may be killed by persistent elevations of corticoids (Sapolsky, Krey, & McEwen, 1985); the hippocampal pyramidal cells have high concentrations of receptors for corticosterone (McEwen, Wallach, & Manius, 1974), as do arcuate neurons for estradiol (Pfaff, 1980). Estradiol treatment of young female rodents induces a hypothalamic-pituitary syndrome that is remarkably similar to spontaneous age changes (see Table 6.1). Similar hypothalamic damage occurs in sheep that fed

TABLE 6.1
Manipulations of Reproductive Aging: The Ovary-Induced
Neuroendocrine Aging Syndrome of Rodents

Markers of Reproductive Aging	Chronic Ovariectomy Delays	Chronic-E2 Accelerates
1. Ovarian cycles lost	Refs. 1, 2	Refs. 3, 4, 5
2. Smaller postovariectomy sensitivity	Ref. 6, 7	Ref. 4
3. Decreased negative feedback sensitivity	Ref. 8	Not known
4. Glial hyperactivity in arcuate nucleus	Ref. 9	Ref. 3
5. Lactotrophe adenomas (a late effect)	Refs. 10, 11	Refs. 12, 13

REFERENCES
1. Aschheim, P. (1965)
2. Felicio, Nelson, Gosden, & Finch (1983)
3. Brawer, Naftolin, Martin, & Sonnenschein (1978)
4. Mobbs et al (1984a)
5. Kawashima, S. (1960)
6. Gee, Flurkey, & Finch (1983)
7. Blake, Elias, & Huffman (1983)
8. Mobbs, C. & Finch, C. (1984b)
9. Schipper, Brawer, Nelson, Felicio, & Finch (1981)
10. Nelson, Felicio, Sinha, & Finch (1980)
11. Mobbs, Gee, & Finch (1984b)
12. Brawer et al (1978)
13. Casanueva et al (1982)

on plant sources with phytoestrogens, which causes "clover disease" (Adams, 1976, 1977, 1983). These effects of estradiol were unexpected, in view of the long-established, perinatal "critical period" in rodents for the "organizing" influence of estradiol on sex differences of hypothalamic circuits (e.g., Gorski, 1968; MacLusky & Naftolin, 1981). The effects of estradiol on the adult rodent brain may contribute to neuroendocrine age changes, since removal of the ovary in young rodents attenuates some aspects of their neuroendocrine aging, including most of the same parameters intensified in young rodents by exposure to estradiol (see Table 6.1). Similarly, adrenalectomy reduces some aspects of hippocampal aging in laboratory rats (Landfield et al., 1978b). These steroid-dependent aging phenomena of rodents suggest that some aspects of brain aging are influenced by endogenous steroids. Over the life span, rodents may experience a cumulative impact of steroids on key neuroendocrine loci (Finch et al., 1980, 1984). The myriad steroids that are now part of our present life, including oral contraceptives, postmenopausal estrogen replacements, anabolic steroids, and anti-inflammatory steroids merit careful evaluation for unexpected, adverse effects. There is little information to determine what, if any, aspects of human brain aging are influenced by steroids, but the biological precedents are now clearly established from studies on lower mammals.

DIRE STRESS

The suggestions that corticoids and other steroids may kill or irreversibly damage nerve cells probably contributes to irreversible aspects of stress on brain function. An extreme of stress effects is the cerebral atrophy of torture victims, characterized by CT scans, which lasts at least six years after the trauma (Jensen et al., 1982). Long-lasting, apparently permanent neuropsychiatric disturbances are observed in these individuals, as well as in survivors of World War II concentration camps (Klonoff, McDougall, Clark, Kramer, & Horgan, 1976; Thygesen, Hermann, & Willanger, 1970). The cortical atrophy and disturbances of memory, emotion, and other behaviors in these victims of dire stress are considered to resemble some dysfunctions also seen in Alzheimer's disease and other age-related dementias (Henry 1986; Jensen et al., 1982). However, despite the behavioral and cognitive similarities to age-related dementias, histologic and biochemical data are not yet available to show if the stress-related dementias share the specific cellular loss, cytological changes, and biochemical deficits observed in Alzheimer's.

Sustained stress can produce physical dysfunctions in young rats like those of aging (e.g., Pare, 1965), a result which is consistent with the concept that senescence results from the accumulation of stress over the life span (Selye & Prioreschi, 1960). The possibility of corticosteroid-induced killing of hippocampal neurons in young rats and the permanent effects of dire stress on humans (cited above) strongly support an interaction of unusual stress with subsequent aging, but need not apply to all types or degrees of stress. A question of great interest in Alzheimer's disease is the possible relationship of hippocampal neuron damage to endogenous corticosteroids and stress. Studies of experimental lesions in rats show that despite initial recovery, deficits can emerge later in life as noted above.

STRESS AND AGE-CORRELATED DEMENTIAS

There is some evidence for possible psychosocial influences on degenerative brain diseases. An exploratory analysis of Norwegian Huntingtonians (Brackenridge, 1979) suggests that occupational stress influences the onset of symptoms in this genetically inevitable disease: A significant difference in mean age of onset separated Huntingtonians in different occupational categories; Huntingtonians with physical occupations (farmers) had a 10-year later age of onset than did a category of sedentary occupations (clerks, draftsman) which may be more anxiety-producing. This striking finding, if extended by subsequent studies, suggests an important potential for psychosocial manipulations of the expression of genotypes which predispose to dementing diseases. Most Huntingtonism cases have an onset during midlife. I have hypothesized that Huntingtonism involves acceleration of age changes in the basal ganglia (Finch, 1980). If the timing of expression of the Huntingtonian genotype with its 100% penetrance can be modified so significantly by stress, then it may also be possible to modify the onset and course of Alzheimer's disease and other age-related dementias. In particular, familial forms of Alzheimer's disease should be carefully studied for possible influences of stress and other psychosocial forces, diet, and drugs. There is also evidence for stressful events causing schizophrenic episodes (Dohrenwend & Egri, 1981).

Another facet of the increased incidence of brain dysfunctions with age may be a greater susceptibility of the elderly to stress. Older surgical patients appear to have a much greater postoperative risk of delirium and other behavioral disturbances (Linn et al., 1953; Bedford, 1955; Gilberstadt & Sako, 1967). Possibly the major, but transient elevations of corticosteroids which occur during general anesthesia and other stresses inflict damage on the brains of elderly patients. Several studies suggest that aging rodents become more sensitive to the effects of estradiol in behavioral tests (Grey, Smith, & Davidson, 1980; Cooper, 1977) and in suppressing LH (Grey, Tennent, Smith, & Davidson, 1980). Also, corticosteroid output during stress can increase in old rats (Hess & Riegle, 1970), and the return to basal corticosteroid levels can be slower (Sapolsky, Krey, & McEwen, 1983). Older humans show greater output of vasopressin in response to blood osmotic pressure changes (Robertson & Rowe, 1980) and greater elevations of plasma norepinephrine in response to standing (Young, Rowe, Pallotta, Sparrow, & Landsberg), 1980). The greater impact of stress with advancing age could result from at least 3 factors: a greater intrinsic cellular susceptibility to damage; a slower return to baseline values which would prolong exposure to corticoids and other possible "stress-neurotoxins"; and, summation of the damage with pre-existing, accumulated neural deficits (Finch et al., 1980).

ADVERSE EFFECTS OF CHRONIC NEUROLEPTICS

The susceptibility to drug side effects increases with age and may interact with brain aging processes. A strong example is that some psychiatric patients, given chronic treatment with neuroleptic (dopaminergic) antagonists develop a permanent motor defect, tardive dyskinesia. This drug-induced disorder is most prevalent among the elderly (e.g., Seide & Muller, 1967; Smith & Baldessarini, 1980). The mechanism is unknown but may involve neuronal loss, since chronic neuroleptic treatment of rats kills striatal neurons according to some reports

(Pakkenberg, Fog, & Nilakantan, 1973; Nielson & Lyon, 1978); also, prolonged neuroleptic treatment (12 months) can cause apparently irreversible increases in the responsiveness of striatal adenylate cyclase to dopamine (Clow, Theodorou, Jenner, & Marsden, 1983). Further examples may be expected from chronic treatment with other neurotropic drugs.

POTENTIAL AMELIORATORS
OF AGING CHANGES IN NEURAL FUNCTIONS

In contrast to the preceding descriptions of adverse influences on brain aging, there are other examples in which neural aging changes can be ameliorated by non-drastic interventions.

Diet

Several examples show a striking potential for the positive influences of nutrition on neural aging processes. The progressive, age-correlated loss of striatal dopamine receptors in laboratory rodents (e.g., Severson & Finch, 1980) is greatly attenuated by dietary restriction (Leven, Handa, Joseph, Ingram, & Roth), 1981) and some motor changes of age are modified (Joseph, Whitaker, Roth, & Ingram, 1983); the mechanism is unknown. Because humans also show a progressive loss throughout adult life in caudate dopaminergic (D-2) binding sites (Severson, Marcusson, Winblad, & Finch, 1982; Morgan, Marcusson, Nyberg, Wester, Winblad, & Finch, 1987), it may be possible to identify nutritional influences on human dopamine receptors as well; for example, by brain-imaging analysis of drug binding sites.

The common hindlimb paralysis of aging rats (Berg, Wolf, & Simms, 1962; Cohen, Anver, Ringler, & Adelman, 1978; Anver, Cohen, Lattuada, & Foster, 1982) that is associated with degeneration of spinal motor neurons (Berg et al., 1962) ("radiculoneuropathy") is also greatly reduced by dietary restriction (Everitt, 1980); mechanism unknown. At the ultrastructural level, old mice can acquire more dendritic processes by supplementing their diets with lecithin (Mervis & Bartus, 1981). Lecithin is a potential contributor to phospholipid membrane constituents, as well as a precursor for acetylcholine.

Chronic restriction of tryptophan may provide another case of dietary influences on brain aging: Such rats, when returned to a normal diet at 2 years, had "youthful" capacity for two brain-mediated functions, thermoregulation (Segall & Timiras, 1975) and fertility (Segall & Timiras, 1976); however, effects of tryptophan restriction could include many peripheral loci, as well as the brain.

These examples suggest that variations in diet may influence neural aging at several levels, including neuronal interactions and neuronal degeneration. A substantial literature already records the extension of life span in rodents by mild dietary restrictions, as well as the reduction of a broad spectrum of degenerative conditions in visceral organs (Osborne, Mendel, & Ferry, 1917; Ross & Bras, 1971; Weindruch & Walford, 1982). Such effects of diet on human longevity in the general case remain to be shown, although there is much evidence that maturity-onset diabetes and some other life-shortening diseases can be partly controlled by diet patterns.

Psychosocial Influences on Brain Aging

The extent to which aging processes in the nervous system can be modified by psychosocial influences is unknown, but a few examples suggest important possibilities. Preliminary reports (Diamond & Connor, 1981; Diamond, 1983) indicate that placement of old rats with young adults increases the thickness of the cerebral cortex and promotes growth of neural processes. Such studies indicate a new set of questions to evaluate the potential responses by different neural systems to the social environment at various stages of aging. The slowed recovery of old rats from brain lesions (e.g. reactive fibre growth in the dentate gyrus; Scheff, Benardo, & Cotman, 1980) suggests age-related limitations of neuronal responsiveness.

SUMMARY

This brief article illustrates the types of influences which can modify age-related changes in the nervous system. These examples suggest that many aspects of brain aging can be influenced by environmental factors and are neither intrinsic nor inevitable. I wonder if there are subtypes of Alzheimer's disease and other age-related dementias in which the onset and course can be extensively modified by psychosocial influences, drugs, or diet. Elucidation of such influences on age-correlated dementias may emerge from the various longitudinal studies of human aging (Migdal, Abeles, & Sherrod, 1981; Shock, 1985).

ACKNOWLEDGMENTS

This research was supported by NIA grants AG 03272 and AG 00117.

REFERENCES

Acheson, A. L., & Zigmond, M. J. (1981). Short- and long-term changes in tyrosine hydroxylase activity in rat brain after subtotal destruction of central noradrenergic neurons. *Journal of Neuroscience, 1*, 493–504.

Adams, N. R. (1976). Pathological changes in the tissues of infertile ewes with clover disease. *Journal of Comparative Pathology, 86*, 29–35.

Adams, N. R. (1977). Morphological changes in the organs of ewes grazing on oestrogenic subterranean clover. *Research in Veterinary Science, 22*, 216–221.

Adams, N. R. (1983). Sexual behavior of ewes with clover disease treated repeatedly with oestradiol benzoate or testosterone proprionate after ovariectomy. *Journal of Reproduction and Fertility, 68*, 113–117.

Anver, M. R., Cohen, B. J., Lattuada, C. P., & Foster, S. J. (1982). Age-associated lesions in barrier-reared male Sprague-Dawley rats. *Experimental Aging Research, 8*, 3–24.

Aschheim, P. (1965). Resultats fournis par la grafte heterochrone des ovarie dans l'etude de la regulation hypothalamus hypophyso-ovarienne de la ratte senile. *Gerontologia, 10*, 65–75.

Bedford, P. D. (1955). Adverse cerebral effects of anaesthesia on old people. *Lancet, 2*(1), 259–263.

Bell, E., Marek, D. L. F., Levinstone, D. S., Merrill, C., Sher, S., Young, I. T., & Eden, M. (1978). Loss of division potential in vitro: Aging or differentiation. *Science, 202*, 1158–1163.

Berg, B. N., Wolf, A., & Simms, H. S. (1962). Degenerative lesions of spinal roots and peripheral nerves in aging rats. *Gerontologia, 6*, 72–80.

Blake, C. A., Elias, K. A., & Huffman, L. J. (1983). Ovariectomy of young adult rats has a sparing effect on the suppressed ability of aged rats to release luteinizing hormone. *Biology of Reproduction, 28*, 575–585.

Brackenridge, C. J. (1979). Relation of occupational stress to the age at onset of Huntington's disease. *Acta Neurologica Scandinavica, 60*, 272–276.

Brawer, J. R., Naftolin, F., Martin, J., & Sonnenschein, C. (1978). Effects of a single injection of estradiol valerate on the hypothalamic arcuate nucleus and on reproductive function in the female rat. *Endocrinology, 103*, 510–512.

Brawer, J. R., & Sonnenschein, C. (1975). Cytopathological effects of estradiol on the arcuate nucleus of the female rat. A possible mechanism for pituitary tumorigenesis. *American Journal of Anatomy, 144*, 57–87.

Casaneuva, F., Cocchi, D., Locatelli, V., Flauto, C., Zambotti, F., Bestetti, F., Rossi, G. L., & Muller, E. (1982). Defective central nervous system dopaminergic function in rats with estrogen-induced pituitary tumors, as assessed by plasma prolactin concentration. *Endocrinology, 110*, 590–599.

Clow, A., Theodorou, A., Jenner, P., & Marsden, C. D. (1980). Cerebral dopamine function in rats following withdrawal from one year of continuous neuroleptic administration. *European Journal of Pharmacology, 63*, 145–147.

Cohen, B. J., Anver, M., Ringler, D., & Adelman, R. C. (1978). The comparative pathology of aging in Sprague-Dawley and Fischer 344 rats. *Federal Proceedings, 37*, 2848–2850.

Cooper, D. L. (1977). Sexual receptivity in aged female rats. Behavioral evidence for increased sensitivity to estrogen. *Hormones and Behavior, 9*, 321.

Diamond, M. C. (1983). The aging rat forebrain: Male-female left-right; environment and lipofuscin. In D. Samuel (Eds.), *Aging of the brain* (Vol. 22, pp. 98–98). New York: Raven Press.

Diamond, M. C., & Connor, J. R., Jr. (1981). A search for the potential of the aging brain. In S. J. Enna, Samorajski, & B. Beer (Eds.), *Brain neurotransmitters and receptors in aging and age-related behaviors* (Vol. 17, pp. 43–58). New York: Raven Press.

Dohrenwend, B. P., & Egri, G. (1981). Recent stressful life events and episodes of schizophrenia. *Schizophrenic Bulletin, 7*, 12–23.

Duncan, D., & Jarvis, W. H. (1943). Observations on repeated regeneration of the facial nerve in cats. *Journal of Comparative Neurology, 79*, 315–325.

Edstrom, J. E., & Eichner, E. (1958). Relation between nucleolar volume and cell body content of ribonucleic acid in supraoptic neurons. *Nature* (London), *181*, 619.

Everitt, A. V., Seedsman, N. J., & Jones, F. (1980). The effects of hypophysectomy and continuous food restriction, begun at ages of 70 and 400 days, on collagen aging, proteinuria, incidence of pathology and longevity in the male rat. *Mechanisms of Aging and Development, 12*, 161–172.

Felicio, L. S., Nelson, J. F., Gosden, R. E., & Finch, C. E. (1983). Restoration of ovulatory cycles by young ovarian grafts in aging mice: Potentiation by long-term ovariectomy decreases with age. *Proceedings of the National Academy of Sciences, 80*, 6076–6080.

Finch, C. E. (1976). The regulation of physiological changes during mammalian aging. *Quarterly Review of Biology, 51*, 49–83.

Finch, C. E. (1980). Relationships of aging changes in the basal ganglia to manifestations of Huntington's chorea. *Annals of Neurology, 7*, 406–411.

Finch, C. E. & Landfield, P. (1985). Neuroendocrine and autonomic aspects of aging. In C. E. Finch & E. L. Schneider (Eds.), *Handbook of the biology of aging* (2nd ed., pp. 79–90). New York: Van Nostrand.

Finch, C. E., Felicio, L. A., Flurkey, K., Gee, D. M., Mobbs, C., Nelson, J. F., & Osterburg, H. H. (1980). Studies in ovarian-hypothalamic-pituitary interactions during reproductive aging in C57BL/6J mice. *Peptides, 1* (Supplement 1), 163–176.

Finch, C. E., Felicio, L. J., Mobbs, C. V., & Nelson, J. F. (19). Ovarian and steroidal influences on neuroendocrine aging processes in female rodents. *Endocrine Reviews, 5*, 467–497.

Florini, J. R., Saito, Y., & Manowitz, E. J. (1973). Effect of age on thyroine-induced cardiac hypertrophy in mice. *Journal of Gerontology, 28*, 293 297.

Gee, D. M., Flurkey, K., & Finch, C. E. (1983). Aging and the regulation of luteinizing hormone in C57BL/6J mice: Impaired elevations after ovariectomy and spontaneous elevations at advanced ages. *Biology of Reproduction, 28*, 598–607.

Gilberstedt, H., & Sako, Y. (1967). Intellectual and personality changes following open-heart surgery. *Archives of General Psychiatry, 16*, 210–214.

Gorski, R. A. (1968). Influence of age on the response to para-natal administration of a low dose of androgen. *Endocrinology, 82*, 1001–1004.

Grey, G. D., Smith, E. R., & Davidson, J. M. (1980). Gonadotropin regulation in middle-aged male rats. *Endocrinology, 107*, 2021–2026.

Grey, G. D., Tennent, B., Smith, E. R., & Davidson, J. M. (1980). Luteinizing hormone regulation and sexual behavior in middle-aged female rats. *Endocrinology, 17*, 187–194.

Hamilton, J. B., Catchpole, H. R., & Hawke, C. C. (1945). Titres of gonadotropins in urine of aged eunuchs. *Journal of Clinical Endocrinology, 5*, 203–209.

Harrison, D. M. (1985). Cell and tissue transplantation: A means of studying the aging process. In C. E. Finch & E. L. Schneider (Eds.), *Handbook of the biology of aging* (2nd ed., pp. 322–356). New York: Van Nostrand.

Hayflick, L., & Moorehead, P. S. (1961). The serial cultivation of human diploid strains. *Experimental Cell Research, 25*, 585–621.

Henry, J. P. (1986). Relation of psychosocial factors to the senile dementias. In M. L. M. Gilhooly, S. H. Zaut, & J. E. Birren (Eds.), *The Dementias: Policy and management* (pp. 38–65). Englewood Cliffs, NJ: Prentice-Hall.

Hess, G. D., & Riegle, G. D. (1970). Adrenocortical responsiveness to stress with ACTH in aging rats. Journal of Gerontology, 25, 354–358.

Hoffman, G. E., & Finch, C. E. (1986). LHRH neurons in female C57BL/6J mice: No loss up to middle-age. *Neurobiology of Aging, 7*, 45–48.

Holland, J. J., Korne, D., & Doyle, M. V. (1973). Analysis of virus replication in aging human fibroblast cultures. *Nature, 245*, 316–318.

Hornsby, P. J., & Gill, G. N. (1978). Characterization of adult bovine adrenocortical cells throughout their life span in tissue culture. *Endocrinology, 102*, 926–936.

Hugin, F., & Verzar, F. (1956). Untersuchungen uber die Arbeitshypertrophie des Herzens bei jungen und alten Ratten. *Pflug. Arch. Ges. Physiol., 262*, 181.

Huxley, T. H. (1896). On the physical basis of life. In *Methods and results, essays*. New York: Appleton-Century.

Ivy, F., Schotter, F., Baudry, M., & Lynch, G. S. (1983). Rapid induction of ceroid formation in rat hippocampus by leupeptin. *Social Neuroscience Abstracts, 9*, 926.

Jensen, T. S., Genefke, I. K., Hyldebrandt, N., Pedersen, H., Petersen, H. D., & Weile, B. (1982). Cerebral atrophy in young torture victims. *New England Journal of Medicine, 307*, 1341.

Joseph, J. A., Whitaker, J., Roth, G. S., & Ingram, D. K. (1983). Life-long dietary restriction affects striatally mediated behavioral responses in aged rats. *Neurobiology of Aging, 4*, 191–196.

Kawashima, S. (1960). Influence of continued injections of sex steroids on the estrous cycle in the adult rat. *Annot. Zool. Japon., 33*, 226–232.

Klonoff, H., McDougall, G., Clark, D., Kramer, P., & Horgan, J. (1976). The neuropsychological, psychiatric, and physical effects of prolonged and severe stress: 30 years later. *Journal of Nervous and Mental Diseases, 163*, 246–252.

Landfield, P. W., Lindsey, J. C., & Lynch, G. (1978a). Apparent acceleration of brain aging pathology by prolonged administration of glucocorticoids. *Social Neuroscience Abstracts, 4*, 350.

Landfield, P. W., Waymire, J. C., & Lynch, G. (1978b). Hippocampal aging and adrenocorticoids: Quantitative considerations. *Science, 202*, 1098–1102.

Leipheimer, P. E., & Gallo, R. V. (1983). Acute and long-term changes in central and pituitary mechanisms regulating pulsatile luteinizing hormone secretion after ovariectomy in the rat. *Neuroendocrinology, 37*, 421–426.

Lesher, S. (1966). Chronic radiation and aging in mice and rats. In P. G. Lindop, & G. Sacher (Eds.), *Radiation and aging* (pp. 183–205). London: Taylor and Francis.

Lesher, S., Fry, S. J. M., & Kohn, H. I. (1961). The influence of age on transit time of cells of mouse intestinal epithelium I Duodenum. *Laboratory Investigation, 10*, 291–300.

Levin, P., Handa, J. K., Joseph, J. A., Ingram, K., & Roth, G. S. (1981). Dietary restriction retards the age-associated loss of rat striatal dopaminergic receptors. *Science, 214*, 561–562.

Lindstedt, S. L., & Calder, W. A., III. (1981). Body size, physiological time, and longevity of homeothermic mammals. *Quarterly Review of Biology, 56*, 1–16.

Linn, L., Kahn, R. L., Coles, R., Cohen, J., Marshall, D., & Weinstein, E. A. (1953). Patterns of behavior disturbance following cataract extraction. *American Journal of Psychiatry, 110*, 281–289.

Lipman, R. D., & Muggleton-Harris, A. L. (1982). Modification of the cataractous phenotype by somatic cell hybridization. *Somatic Cell Genetics, 8*, 791–800.

MacLusky, N. J., & Naftolin, F. (1981). Sexual differentiation of the central nervous system. *Science, 211*, 1294–1303.

Man, E. H., Sandhouse, M. E., Burg, J., & Fisher, G. H. (1983). Accumulation of D-aspartic acid with age in human brain. *Science, 220*, 1407–1408.

Mann, D. M. A., & Yates, P. O. (1982). Is the loss of cerebral cortical choline acetyltransferase activity in Alzheimer's disease due to degeneration of ascending cholinergic nerve cells? *Journal of Neurology, Neurosurgery, and Psychiatry, 45*, 936–943.

Mann, D. M. A., & Yates, P. O. (1983). Possible role of neuromelanin in the pathogenesis of Parkinson's disease. *Mechanisms of Aging Development, 21*, 193–203.

Masters, P. M., Bada, J. L., & Zigler, J. S., Jr. (1975). Aspartic acid racemization in heavy molecular weight crystallins and water-soluble protein from normal human lens and cataracts. *Proceedings of the National Academy of Sciences* (U.S.), *75*, 1204–1208.

Masters-Helfman, P., & Bada, J. L. (1975). Aspartic acid racemization in tooth enamel from living humans. *Proceedings of the National Academy of Sciences* (U.S.), *72*, 2891–2894.

McEwen, B. S., Wallach, G., & Manius, C. (1974). Corticosterone binding to hippocampus: Immediate and delayed influences of the absence of adrenal secretion. *Brain Research, 70*, 321–334.

Mervis, R. F., & Bartus, R. T. (1981). Modulation of pyramidal cell dendritic spine population in aging mouse neocortex: Role of dietary choline. *Journal of Neuropathology and Experimental Neurology, 40*, 313.

Migdal, S., Abeles, R. P., & Sherrod, L. R. (1981). *An inventory of longitudinal studies of middle and old age.* New York: Social Science Research Council.

Mobbs, C. V., Flurkey, K., Gee, D. M., Yamamoto, K., Sinha, Y. N., & Finch, C. E. (1984a). Estradiol-induced anovulatory syndrome in female C57BL/6J mice: Age-like neuroendocrine, but not ovarian, impairments. *Biology of Reproduction, 30*, 556–563.

Mobbs, C. V., Gee, D. M., & Finch, C. E. (1984b). Reproductive senescence in female C57BL/6J mice: Ovarian impairments and neuroendocrine impairments that are partially reversible and delayable by ovariectomy. *Endocrinology, 115*, 1653–1662.

Monagle, R. D., & Brody, H. (1974). The effects of age upon the main nucleus of the inferior olive in the human. *Journal of Comparative Neurology, 155*, 61–66.

Morgan, D. G., Marcusson, J. O., Nyberg, P., Wester, P., Winblad, B., & Finch, C. E. (1987). Divergent changes in D-1 and D-2 dopamine binding sites in human basal ganglia during normal aging. *Society of Neurobiology of Aging.*

Nelson, J. F., Felicio, L. S., Sinha, Y. N., & Finch, C. E. (1980). An ovarian role in the spontaneous pituitary tumorigenesis. *The Gerontologist* (abstract), *20*(5, Part II), 171.

Nielson, E. B., & Lyon, M. (1978). Evidence for cell loss in corpus striatum after long-term treatment with a neuroleptic drug (fluphenthixol) in rats. *Psychopharmacology, 59*, 85–89.

Osborne, T. B., Mendel, L. B., & Ferry, E. L. (1917). The effect of retardation of growth upon the breeding period and duration of life in rats. *Science, 45*, 294.

Pakkenberg, H., Fog, H. F., & Nilakantan, B. (1973). The long-term effect of perphenazine enanthate on the rat brain. Some metabolic and anatomical observations. *Psychopharmacology* (Berlin), *29*, 329–336.

Pare, W. P. (1965). The effect of chronic environmental stress on premature aging in the rat. *Journal of Gerontology, 20*, 78–84.

Pasinetti, G., Morgan, D. G., & Finch, C. D. (in prep). Compensatory responses to cholingergic lesions in rat brain.

Pedata, F., Lo Conte, G., Sorbi, S., Marconcini-Pepeu, J., & Pepeu, G. (1982). Changes in high affinity choline uptake in rat cortex following lesions of the magnocellular forebrain nuclei. *Brain Research, 233*, 359–367.

Pfaff, D. W. (1980). *Estrogens and brain function.* New York: Springer-Verlag.

Poskanzer, D. C., & Schwab, R. S. (1961). Studies in the epidemiology of Parkinson's disease predicting its disappearance as a major clinical entity by 1980. *Transactions of the American Neurological Association, 86*, 234–235.

Robertson, G. L., & Rowe, J. (1980). The effect of aging or neurohypophyseal function. *Peptides, 1*(Suppl. 1), 159–162.

Ross, M. H., & Bras, G. (1971). Lasting effect of early caloric restriction on prevention of neoplasms in the rat. *Journal of the National Cancer Institute, 47*, 1095–1113.

Rubner, M. (1908). Probleme des Wachstums en der Lebendauer. *Mitt. inn. Med. Kinderheilk. Wein, 7*(Beil. 9), 58.

Sacher, G. A., & Duffy, P. H. (1979). Genetic relation of life span to metabolic rate for inbred mouse strains and their hybrids. *Federal Proceedings, 38*, 184–188.

Sapolsky, R. M., Krey, L. C., & McEwen, B. S. (1983). The adrenocortical stress response in the aged male rat: Impairment of recovery from stress. *Experimental Gerontology, 18*, 55–64.

Sapolsky, R. M., Krey, L. C., & McEwen, B. S. (1985). Prolonged glycocortical exposure reduces hippocampal neuron number: Implications for aging. *Journal of Neuroscience, 5*, 1221–1226.

Sarkar, D. K., Gottschall, P. E., & Meites, J. (1982). Damage to hypothalamic dopaminergic neurons is associated with development of prolactin-secreting pituitary tumors. *Science, 218*, 684–686.

Scaglia, H., Medina, H. M., Pinto-Ferreira, A. L., Vasquez, G., Gual, C., & Perez-Palacios, G. (1976). Pituitary LH and FSH secretion and responsiveness in women of old age. *Acta Endocrinologica, 81*, 673–679.

Schallert, T. (1983). Sensorimotor impairment and recovery of function in brain-damaged rats: Reappearance of symptoms during old age. *Behavioral Neuroscience, 97*, 159–164.

Scheff, S. W., Benardo, L. S., & Cotman, C. W. (1980). Decline in reactive fibre growth in the dentate gyrus of aged rats compared to young adult rats following entorhinal cortex removal. *Brain Research, 199*, 21–38.

Schipper, H., Brawer, J. R., Nelson, J. F., Felicio, L. S., & Finch, C. E. (1981). The role of gonads in the histologic aging of the hypothalamic arcuate nucleus. *Biology of Reproduction, 25*, 413–419.

Segall, P. E., & Timiras, P. S. (1975). Age-related changes in thermo-regulatory capacity of tryptophan-deficient rats. *Federal Proceedings, 34*, 83–85.

Segall, P. E., & Timiras, P. S. (1976). Pathophysiologic findings after chronic tryptophan deficiency in rats: A model for delayed growth and aging. *Mechanisms of Aging and Development, 5*, 109–124.

Seide, H., & Muller, H. (1967). Choreiform movements as side effects of phenothiazine medication in geriatric patients. *Journal of the American Geriatric Society, 15*, 517–522.

Selye, H., & Prioreschi, P. (1960). Stress theory of aging. In N. W. Shock (Ed.), *Aging: Some social and biological aspects* (pp. 261–272). Washington, DC: American Association for the Advancement of Science.

Severson, J. A., & Finch, C. E. (1980). Reduced dopaminergic binding during aging in the rodent striatum. *Brain Research, 139*, 109–177.

Severson, J. A., Marcusson, J., Winblad, B., & Finch, C. E. (1982). Age-correlated loss of dopaminergic binding sites in human basal ganglia. *Journal of Neurochemistry, 39*, 1623–1631.

Shock, N. W. (1985). Longitudinal studies of aging in humans. In C. E. Finch & E. L. Schneider (Eds.), *Handbook of the biology of aging* (2nd ed., pp. 721–743). New York: Van Nostrand.

Smith, J. M., & Baldessarini, R. J. (1980). Changes in prevalence, severity and recovery in tardive dyskinesia with age. *Archives of General Psychiatry, 37*, 1368–1373.

Thygesen, P., Hermann, K., & Willanger, R. (1970). Concentration camp survivors in Denmark. *Danish Medical Bulletin, 17*, 65–108.

Toth, S. E. (1968). The origin of lipofuscin age pigments. *Experimental Gerontology, 3*, 19–30.

Van Peenen, H. J., & Gerstl, B. (1962). Arteriosclerotic massive hypertrophy of the heart. *Journal of the American Geriatric Society, 10*, 505–508.

Watson, W. E. (1968). Observations on the nucleolar and total cell body nucleic acid of injured nerve cells. *Journal of Physiology, 196*, 655–676.

Weindruch, R., & Walford, R. L. (1982). Dietary restriction in mice beginning at 1 year of age: Effect on life span and spontaneous cancer incidence. *Science, 215*, 1415–1418.

Wenk, G. L., & Olton, D. S. (1984). Recovery of neurocortical choline acetyltransferase activity following ibotenic acid injection into the nucleus basalis of Meynert in rats. *Brain Research, 293*, 184–186.

Yates, F. E. (in press). Senescence from the aspect of physical stability. In F. E. Yates (Ed.), *Self-organizing systems*. New York: Plenum Press.

Young, J. B., Rowe, J. W., Pallotta, J. A., Sparrow, D., & Landsberg, L. (1980). Enhanced plasma norepinephrine response to upright posture and oral glucose administration in elderly human subjects. *Metabolism, 29*, 532–539.

7

IMMUNITY AND AGING IMMUNOLOGIC AND BEHAVIORAL PERSPECTIVES

Norman S. Braveman*
Physiology of Aging Branch
National Institute on Aging

This chapter reviews what is known about the aging immune system. I take the point of view that the study of the aging immune system, as well as of the immune system in general, should be undertaken by viewing the immune system as part of an interactive network of systems whose job it is to maintain homeostasis (i.e., to help the organism make adjustments to environmental changes). Traditionally, this network has included the CNS and the endocrine system and the environmental perturbations have, for the most part, included stimuli that are external to the organism. However, there is no apparent reason why the network cannot be expanded to include each and every system of the organism, ranging from the major histocompatibility complex in man (or the HLA system in mice), which controls the genetic expression of lymphocytes, to the cardiovascular system which, in part, transports peripheral blood lymphocytes to various parts of the body. Nor is there any reason why the stimuli that trigger the action of the network cannot include the introduction of antigenic material. The important point is that, when viewed from this perspective, the immune system not only helps the organism to adapt to environmental changes stemming from the presence of foreign molecules, but it also provides feedback to other parts of the larger network which, in turn, plays important roles in adaptation to environmental change.

---

*Present Address: Executive Secretary; Clinical Trials Review Committee; Review Branch; National Heart, Lung and Blood Institute; Westwood Building; Room 550; Bethesda, MD 20205.

The immune system is one of the most complex and pervasive systems of the body. It functions to help protect against challenges from more than one million different molecular species of antigens, and it must meet these challenges in a timely manner with substantially fewer numbers of cells than the antigens which it must recognize—all the while being able to discriminate between those antigens that are produced by normal body tissues (i.e., self) and those that are not (i.e., non-self). In accomplishing this rather formidable task, the immune system must also regulate its own activities by "turning on" and "turning off" various functions. In addition to providing protection against foreign antigens, recent evidence suggests that the immune system may also play a homeostatic role similar to that of the neuroendocrine system. In this role, signals to and from the immune system are crucial to maintaining homeostasis and, therefore, normal functioning of the various organ systems of the body.

The purpose of the present chapter is to review what is known about age-related changes in the protective and the system-interactive aspects of the immune system. This will be accomplished first by examining some basic concepts from immunology and then by reviewing data which give clues about the kinds of functional changes that occur with advancing age. In examining what is known about the aging immune system, particuluar attention will be paid to the possible contributions of the behavioral sciences in furthering our understanding of the impact that aging has on immune function. As background for the chapter we will begin with a very brief and simplified overview of the various parts and functions of the immune system.

COMPONENTS OF THE IMMUNE SYSTEM

The primary or central organs of the immune system consist of bone marrow (which generates stem cells and B lymphocytes in mammals), the thymus gland (in which stem cells differentiate into T lymphocytes), and the bursa of Fabricus in avians (in which stem cells differentiate into B lymphocytes). The spleen and lymph nodes are considered to be peripheral or secondary organs. They contain lymphocytes, plasma cells, and structural cells. Another important cell type of the immune system is the macrophage. These are ubiquitous phagocytic cells which also function to present antigen (i.e., substances that elicit immune responses) to lymphocytes. It is through the interacton of these cells that immune responses are initiated. Both of these cell types, macrophages and lymphocytes, are derived from multipotent stem cells in the bone marrow. These cells, in turn, originate in the yolk sac and, during embryogenesis, migrate to the liver.

The immune response is stimulated by molecules called antigens which, in most instances, are foreign to those that comprise the normal tissues of the organism. Antigens can be soluble or particulate, but the only requirement for a substance to be an antigen is that it be capable of eliciting an immune response. Antigenic stimulation leads to the generation of functional effector B and T cells or to a tolerant state which prevents further responses from occurring. The effector cells that are generated by antigen-stimulated B cells are plasma cells which synthesize and secrete various types of immunoglobulin molecules called antibodies. These antibodies are capable of combining with the antigen and, along with other factors (e.g., complement) and cells (e.g., macrophages), provide protection against infectious agents. T cells, on the other hand, are transformed into several different types of effector cells following antigenic stimulation. Some of these directly lyse foreign cells while other T cell types synthesize and secret hormone-like substances called lymphokines which are important regulatory products in the immune response. According to the clonal selection theory, lymphocytes, once stimulated, produce progeny, some of which deal with the current antigenic challenge while the remaining ones (memory cells) prepare to deal with subsequent challenges.

Two important characteristics of both cellular and humoral immune responses are the specificity of the response and the fact that the response exhibits characteristics which suggest that it "remembers" past encounters with antigens. Specificity refers to the fact that during the immune response antibodies are directed to the unique determinants of antigens and will react only with those specific determinants. The specificity of the relationship between antibody and antigen is determined by the chemical structure and binding characteristics of the antigen and antibody molecules. So it is possible for an antibody to react with an antigen that has a chemically compatible structure. If the chemical structures of two antigens are similar enough, then it is possible for a "cross-reactivity" to occur between a single antibody and the two antigens. Cross-reactivity is used for practical purposes in immunization protocols. For example, the antigenic determinants for smallpox and cowpox appear to be similar enough that antibodies produced against cowpox following immunization are also effective against smallpox antigens. On the other hand, immunization against smallpox does not appear to have any effect on host susceptibility to mumps since the antigenic determinants of the mumps and smallpox virus molecules are chemically dissimilar and, therefore, not cross-reactive.

Immunologic memory refers to the fact that, following the first exposure to an antigen, the immune system is capable of responding at a faster rate, greater amounts of antibody or effector cells are produced, and the antibody has a higher affinity for the antigen. The net effect of immunologic memory is that second and subsequent challenges are dealt with more effectively and efficiently than primary challenges. In part, immunologic memory is a consequence of clonal selection and the expansion of those lymphocytes that contain receptors or determinants for antigens that caused the initial immune response. It is this important characteristic of the immune system that underlies the protective effects of immunization.

THE ROLE OF THE THYMUS

As noted above, the thymus is one of the primary organs of the immune system. It also appears to play a central role in some of the aging changes that occur in immune functioning. The thymus in humans is located at the base of the neck. Cells from the bone marrow migrate to the cortex of the thymus, differentiate, and become immunocompetent T (for thymus-derived) cells. The differentiation process appears to rely on polypeptide hormones which are synthesized by the endocrine portion of the thymus. As a class, they are referred to as thymic hormones. However, individual polypeptides have been characterized and sequenced and are referred to as thymic humoral factor (Tranin et al., 1975), thymopoietin (Goldstein, 1975), facteur thymique serique (Bach, Dardene, Pleu, & Bach, 1975), or thymosin and its various synthetic polypeptides (Goldstein & Zatz, 1981).

The cells that are processed by the thymus play varied roles in the immune system. On the one hand, T cells can help regulate or modulate the activities of other T cells as well as the antibody-producing B cells. These regulatory cells can either enhance (helper T cells) or decrease (suppressor T cells) the action of other immunocompetent cells. The second function fulfilled by T cells involves cellular immune responses. In this capacity, cytotoxic T cells (i.e., killer cells) lyse other cells, such as tumors, by direct contact between the two cells. Other effector T cells, which produce substances called lymphokines, are involved in delayed hypersensitivity reactons (e.g., inflammatory reactions elicited by an antigen 24 to 48 hours after contact with the immunogen), contact hypersensitivity (e.g., similar to delayed hypersensitivity but occurring much more rapidly), and resistance to certain bacterial infections (e.g., *Mycobacterium tuberculosis, Salmonella typohsa*). It is important to note that these many and varied functions of T cells are carried out by cells that are all processed by the thymus but which have distinctive physiological and functional characteristics.

Research has shown that age-related changes in the thymus are correlated with many aging changes in immune functioning. One of the earliest descriptions of aging changes in the structure of the thymus was reported by Boyd (1932). She examined physiological changes in thymuses obtained from deceased patients through 90 years of age. Her findings showed that the thymus begins to involute or atrophy at about the age of sexual maturity. Involution, which was characterized by replacement of normal tissue by connective tissue and fat, appeared to be complete by 45–50 years. One concomitant of a shrinking thymus with increasing age appears to be a loss of functional capacity of the organ and the cells that it processes. In an early study, Hirokawa and Makinodan (1975) showed that thymuses grafted to neonatally thymectomized mice restored the T-cell population if the donor of the thymus graft was young. If, on the other hand, the donor was old, there were few, if any, restorative effects of the graft on the T-cell population.

The specific defect in the thymuses from old donors appears to be associated with the ability of the organ to support differentiation of immature lymphocytes into mature or immunocompetent cells. However, it is possible that the defect is not in the thymus itself but in some other aspect of the processing apparatus, for example, a pre- or post-thymic component. It is known, for example, that fewer stem cells enter the thymus with increasing age. At the same time, the percentage of *immature* lymphocytes (i.e., undifferentiated cells) within the thymus (Singh & Singh, 1979) and within the blood plasma of humans (Moody et al., 1981) *increases* with age. So, it appears that even though fewer cells are being made available to the thymus from bone marrow for differentiation, more immature cells are present in peripheral blood. Apparently, the decline in mature T cells present in peripheral blood is caused by age-related changes in the ability of the thymus to modify its capacity to generate functional T cells and is not a function of age-related changes in the availability of stem cells. The exact cause of the decline in differentiated lymphocytes is not known but may be related to corresponding age-related changes in the synthesis of thymic hormones. For example, circulating levels of thymopoietin in humans begins to decline at about 30 years of age and reaches levels that are undetectable by about 60 years (Weksler, 1981). It is possible that this decline in thymic hormone levels is responsible for the decline in differentiated T cells found in aged individuals.

Although the thymus is considered to be an integral organ of the immune system, there is ample evidence that it also plays an important role in the neuroendocrine system. Rebar and colleagues (Rebar, Mijake, Low, & Goldstein, 1981), for example, have shown that thymosin interacts with hypothalamic cells to induce the release of leutenizing hormone releasing factor from cultured pituitary cells. Moreover, in an early study Pierpaoli and Besedovsky (1975), using congenitally athymic mice, showed that a functioning thymus was necessary during development in order to produce a functional hypothalamic-pituitary axis at maturity. Similarly, it has been shown that a normally functioning thymus is important in the initiation of follicle growth in the rat ovary (Linten-Moore, 1977). More recenly, Hall and colleagues (Hall, McGillis, & Goldstein, 1984), building on the earlier work of Besedovsky and Sorkin (1977), have provided a detailed analysis of the pathways involved in the activation of neuroendocrine pathways by the thymus, specifcally by thymosin. These examples show that the thymus is critical to other functions as well as to the processing of stem cells from bone marrow into immunocompetent T cells. However, one might conclude that there is a unidirectional relationship between the thymus and the endocrine/neuroendocrine system. This is not the case, and there is ample evidence that extra-immunologic factors may influence thymic functioning. On the one hand, we have already noted that thymic hormones are crucial in the normal development of T lymphocytes. It also appears that growth hormones (e.g., Arrenbrecht & Sorkin, 1973) and sex hormones (Lahita, 1982; Talal, Dauphinee, & Roubinien, 1981) play an important role in this process as well. Further, it is known that the thymus is innervated by fibers from the sympathetic (Williams et al., 1981) and parasympathetic (Bulloch & Moore, 1980) arms of the nervous system. Unpublished findings by Markesberry (personal communication, 1984) suggest the presence of large perivascular seritonergic nerves composed of both myelinated and unmyelinated fibers near the surface of the thymus. That the thymus is innervated by these nerves is suggested by the finding that some thymic cells contain cytoplasmic reaction products to serotonin. Interestingly, older animals appear to exhibit larger amounts of endoneurial fibrous tissue around these fibers when compared to younger animals.

Thus it appears that there are two-way connections between the thymus and the endocrine and nervous systems. In addition to the age-related anatomical changes that occur in the thymus itself, it appears that some of the neurologic and/or endocrinologic connections may also exhibit structural and/or functional changes with increasing age which, in turn, can influence immune function. Equally as important, however, are the concomitant age-associated life events that appear to have an effect on immune function via the neuroendocrine-thymus axis (e.g., retirement, loss of a spouse or other close friend(s), progressive isolation from familiar environments, prolonged medication, and other "stressful" events). These "behavioral" events may influence the ultimate production of immunocompetent lymphocytes by modifying the production and/or action of the thymic hormones. However, until the functional connections between the behavioral events and the endocrine/CNS mediators as well as between these physiologic systems and behavioral events are delineated, the relationship between behavioral events and immune function must remain speculative. Similarly, additional research is required in order to document any causal relationship between changes in immune status that might, via endocrine or CNS pathways, modify behavior.

CELLULAR IMMUNITY

It has already been noted that one important consequence of thymic involution is a decline in the differentiation of mature T cells. As noted previously, T cells are both modulators and effectors of the immune system, and both of these functions appear to be influenced by age-related changes in the thymus. In this section we will focus on aging changes in cellular immunity, leaving the discussion of regulatory changes for a later section.

In one of the earliest studies on the aging immune system it was observed that hypersensitivity reactions, which are T-cell mediated, were modified in the elderly so that when individuals were sensitized to dinitrochlorobenzene and then challenged with the same antigen, 30 percent of those over 70 years failed to respond to the antigen while fewer than 5 percent of subjects under 70 failed to respond (Waldorf, Wilkens, & Decker, 1968). Another T-cell deficit in elderly individuals can be seen in the graft vs. host reaction. This reaction is caused by the transplantation of immunocompetent T cells to a host that is unable to reject the cells and thus becomes the target of attack by these cells. Graft rejection involves an intricate series of immune reactions, ending in the generation of cytotoxic T cells. Old mice have been shown to be deficient in the graft vs. host reaction (Friedman, Keiser, & Globerson, 1974), apparently because they are unable to produce sufficient numbers of cytotoxic T cells (Bach, 1979). Interestingly, incubation of T cells from old animals in thymic hormone preparations restored the ability of these cells to mount an in vitro rejection response (Friedman et al., 1974). It is findings such as these that lead to the conclusion that age-related changes in thymic hormones are responsible for the age-related functional deficits in cell-mediated immunity.

A third area of T-cell deficiency that may have important clinical implications for the elderly involves the susceptibility to infectious diseases. Epidemiological studies show an increasing prevalence of infectious diseases in both aging humans and animals. Some studies suggest that, at least in older animals, this may result from interference with the generation of cytotoxic T responses. The increased susceptibility to infectious agents in older subjects appears not to be the result of changes in the number of cytotoxic cells or the result of a decline in the precursors of these cells. Rather, it appears to be caused by a deficit in the production by helper T cells of a hormone-like substance called interleukin-2 (IL-2) which promotes differentiation and proliferation of cytotoxic T cells (Miller & Stuttman, 1981; Stuttman, 1981).

Other animal studies involving the infectious agent *Listeria monocytogenes* reveal that aged mice have a diminished ability to resist infections from this source. Peak protective T-cell production following infection does not appear to differ between young and old mice. Moreover, young and old mice appear to produce equivalent numbers of T cells. However, individual T cells from young animals transfer at least a thousandfold more protection against the infectious agent than do cells from old animals. Also, mediator T cells from young animals are 10 times as efficient in transferring adoptive immunity as are cells from old animals (Patel, 1981). Thus, the effects of aging on this aspect of immune functioning appear, in some as yet unspecified way, to reduce the effectiveness of individual cells to provide protection against infectious agents.

The basis for many of these cellular immune reactions is the proliferation or recruitment of sufficient numbers of immunocompetent cells. Generally speaking, the proliferative responses of T cells are studied in vitro using lymphocyte activation techniques. These techniques involve the addition of mitogens to lymphocytes in culture. Mitogens are substances that cause DNA synthesis and hence cellular proliferation in lymphocytes even without the presence of an antigen. Research has shown that several of these mitogens are relatively cell-specific in that they stimulate one type of lymphocyte (e.g., T cells) but not the other (e.g., B cells). Mitogens such as phytohemagglutinin (PHA), concanavilin

A (ConA), and antithymocyte globulin (ATG) primarily stimulate T cells and are used to examine, experimentally, the capacity of lymphocytes to synthesize DNA and, hence, to divide in much the same way as they would when challenged in vivo by an antigen.

Results of studies with mitogens reveal that lymphocytes from old donors (both humans and animals) are impaired in terms of their ability to proliferate. This impairment is not caused by the inability of these cells to bind the mitogen (which would effectively reduce the ability of the mitogen to stimulate the cell to divide) in that there appears to be no difference in the number and affinity of receptors for PHA on lymphocytes from young and old animals. Yet samplings of cells from old donors produce only 20 to 50 percent as many mitogen responsive cells as are obtained from young human donors (Inkeles, Innes, & Kuntz, 1977). Further, the capacity of the responsive cells to divide sequentially is reduced in older individuals. Hefton and colleagues (Hefton, Darlington, & Casazza, 1980), for example, have shown that after 96 hours in culture with PHA the number of lymphocytes from old individuals that divided for the first time was equivalent to that of young subjects. There was, however, a substantial reduction in the number of cells obtained from old donors dividing for a second and third time. Specifically, the number of cells dividing for the second time in old individuals was approximately 50 percent of the amount found in young individuals, while the number of cells from old donors dividing for the third time was only approximately 25 percent of that observed in cells from young individuals. The net effect is that old individuals produce fewer immunocompetent T cells in response to mitogenic stimulation because of a deficit in the proliferative capacity of these cells. In a sense, the cells from old donors appear to stop dividing or proliferating sooner than lymphocytes from young donors.

There are many possible reasons for the proliferative defect in T cells from old donors. One of them, which I will refer to as the cellular energy hypothesis, states that as cells age, an essential defect in the energy centers of lymphocytes occurs. These energy centers, called mitochondria, are long, thin organelles found in the cytoplasm of almost all cells. They recover energy from sugars, fatty acids, and amino acids and are also involved in the formation of a waste product, urea, which is excreted by the kidney. The energy formed by the mitochondria is stored in the form of adenosine triphosphate (ATP). According to the cellular energy hypothesis, age-related defects in the proliferation of lymphocytes is caused by parallel age-related defects in the energy function of mitochondria. Verity and colleagues (Verity, Tam, Cheung, Mock, & Walford, 1983), for example, have shown that ATP in lymphocytes from young donors increases sharply between 24 and 48 hours after stimulation by PHA. Similar levels of ATP in lymphocytes from old donors are not reached until 72 hours after stimulation. These investigators also reported that the source of ATP in both young and old lymphocytes was mitochondrial oxidative phosphorylation. These findings confirm those reported by Chapman and colleagues (Chapman, Zaun, & Gracy, 1981) who suggested that impaired phosphorylation could be the cause of the decreased energy status of old lymphocytes. Furthermore, Verity et al. note that there is a chain of events, beginning with the mitogen-induced expansion of ATP pools and ending with DNA synthesis, which may be impaired in lymphocytes from old donors. As noted earlier, DNA synthesis is an essential step in the proliferation of lymphocytes. Thus anything that interferes with DNA synthesis would, in turn, interfere with the ability of lymphocytes to proliferate.

A second explanation of impaired proliferation of aged lymphocytes, which is not totally unrelated to the cellular energy hypothesis, involves the replicative capacity of DNA in old lymphocytes. It is known, for example, that DNA from old lymphocytes is more susceptible to damage from environmental factors (e.g., tritiated thymidine) than the DNA from young individuals. Tritiated thymidine, which is typically used to measure the proliferative capacity of cells, can cause genetic damage and cell cycle arrest in lymphocytes from old but not from young donors (Staiano-Coico et al., 1983). The basis for the greater susceptibility to DNA damage in old than in young cells is not known. However, it may be related to aging changes in cellular calcium ion transport. In particular, calcium ions are known to play an important role in the mitogenesis of lymphocytes, including those from old donors. For example, cells from old donors appear to be more sensitive to calcium chelators, require greater calcium supplementation to restore proliferative responsiveness, and are more susceptible to the disruptive effects of a calcium channel blocker than lymphocytes from young donors (Blistein-Wellinger & Deinenstein, 1978; Kennes, Hubert, & Broher, 1981). It may be that more general age-related perturbations in calcium metabolism are responsible for the specific proliferative deficits observed in lymphocytes from old donors. In other words, the proliferative changes of lymphocytes that have been noted with increasing age could, in turn, be caused by more general age-related changes in calcium regulation, which we noted earlier is controlled to a certain extent by the mitochondria. It has been suggested elsewhere (e.g., Khachaturian, 1984) that changes in calcium transport may be the cause of aging changes in brain cells. According to this hypothesis, the action or the effect of calcium ions and calcium modulators, which are important links between hormones and intracellular activities (including cell metabolism and, in the present case, perhaps DNA replication), may change with age. Although speculative, this hypothesis has the benefit of being generally applicable to cells of all physiological systems and therefore provides a framework for future research on the aging immune system in which the immune system is viewed as an integral part of an interactive and interdependent network of systems whose combined action maintains the homeostasis of the entire organism.

Whatever the cause of the age-related changes in proliferative capacity, it is clear that cells from aged subjects show proliferative deficits which, in turn, appear to have an important impact on the ability of aged individuals to mount an immune response to antigenic challenge. Some of the deficits that interfere with a normal immune response may result from age-related changes in other systems (e.g., changes in calcium ion transport); others may be caused by changes intrinsic to the immune system; and still others may be caused by factors stemming from behavioral events that are mediated by various physiological systems. It is clear that much additional research is required in order to delineate the various possibilities.

HUMORAL IMMUNITY

The humoral arm of the immune system consists of lymphocytes referred to as B cells. They are so named because in avians, where they were first identified, they differentiate in the bursa of Fabricus. In mammals it is thought that these cells mature in a bone marrow equivalent on the bursa. The main function of B cells is to produce protein molecules called antibodies. Mature B cells differentiate into antibody-secreting cells upon stimulation by an antigen. Antigenic stimulation also causes these cells to proliferate. Thus the net result of antigenic stimulation is twofold: (a) the secretion of antibodies that deal with the immediate challenge; and (b) the acquisition of immunologic memory in the form of a pool of mature lymphocytes which allows the organism to deal effectively with future challenges.

In humans there are five classes of immunoglobulins (Ig) that function as antibodies by combining with antigen. The five major classes of Ig are designed as IgG, IgA, IgM, IgD and IgE. The differences among the five classes are dependent on the structure of part (i.e., the heavy chain) of the molecule. In addition, each of the Ig classes performs a specific set of biologic functions. IgG, for example, can (a) neutralize the soluble exotoxins produced by bacteria, (b) agglutinate bacteria, viruses, and other foreign substances, (c) coat bacteria in order to enhance the phagocytic action of other cells (i.e., opsonize the bacteria), and (d) activate the complement system to promote the lysis of certain strains of gram-negative bacteria. IgM, on the other hand, not only can (a) neutralize toxins, (b) agglutinate bacteria, and (c) activate the complement system but, along with IgD, it is also the major antigen receptor expressed on the surface of B cells. IgA is similar in its biologic activity to IgM, but it does not serve as an antigenic receptor on the surface of B cells. Finally, IgE, because of certain unique properties, can combine with mast cells and basophils at the same time that it combines with antigen. This causes the release of substances such as histamine from the mast cell or basophil. By altering the permeability of small blood vessels, histamine allows antibodies of various classes and phagocytic cells to accumulate at the site where the antigen was encountered. Most IgE-mediated reactions involve exposure of the skin and/or mucosal surfaces to antigens as in immediate hypersensitivity reactions.

The effects of aging on humoral immunity can be both subtle and pervasive. On the one hand, it is known that neither the total number of B lymphocytes nor the total concentration of serum Ig changes with age. The distribution of the various Ig classes, however, does appear to change with age so that IgA and IgG increase in older humans while IgM decreases (Hallgren, Buckley, Gilbertson, & Yunis, 1973). In addition, the concentration of antibody to sheep erythrocytes and salmonella flagellin is lower in the elderly (Paul & Bunnell, 1952; Roberts-Thomson, Whittinghaus, & Youngchaiyud, 1974). Furthermore, there is an age-related decline in IgM- and IgG-producing plaque-forming cells in mice following in vivo immunization with sheep red blood cells (Friedman & Globerson, 1978). In aging rodents, a decline in antibody response with age has been noted following an initial (primary) antigenic challenge but not following subsequent (secondary) challenges (Mackinodan & Kay, 1980). Finally, it has been reported that a tenfold higher dose of antigen is necessary to produce a maximal antibody response in old mice than in young ones (Makinodan & Adler, 1975), corresponding to the observation cited earlier that, on a per-cell basis, cells from old donors appear to provide less protective capacity against infectious agents than do those from young donors.

Cells from aged mice show greater heterogeneity with respect to surface Ig. Populations of B cells from old mice have fewer cells with high-density Ig, and the rate of shedding surface Ig is slower than in young mice (Woda & Feldman, 1979; Rosenberg, Gilman, & Feldman, 1982). It appears that, as in other types of cells, the microviscosity of the B-cell membrane is increased with increasing age so that the movement of the membrane molecules to one region of the cell surface after binding to antigen (i.e., capping) is impaired in cells from old donors. This process of capping appears to be a crucial step in mounting an effective humoral immune response by concentrating the antibody-antigen complex at one point on the cell. Interference with this process ultimately leads to a less effective humoral immune response.

B cells from old donors exhibit some of the same proliferative defects that have been observed in T cells. Fewer B cells from old donors are activated by mitogens such as lipopolysaccharide (Segre & Segre, 1976) or from anti-Ig reagents (Rosenberg et al., 1982). There is a decrease in the number of activated cells from old donors that pass successfully through the cell cycle, and fewer progeny are generated by those cells that do complete the cycle, presumably because of a faster return of mature cells to the resting phase of the cell cycle (Joncourt, Kristensen, & deWeck, 1982).

Another striking change in the humoral arm of the aging immune system is the increase in autoantibodies (i.e., antibodies to self-antigens). Recently it has been speculated that some of the diseases of the elderly (e.g., senile dementia, adult-onset diabetes and/or glucose intolerance, and osteoporosis) may result from specific autoreactive antibodies (e.g., to brain cells, to islet cells of the pancreas or to insulin receptors on various cells, and to bone cells, respectively). As we shall see in a subsequent section, there appears to be an age-associated increase in brain-reactive antibodies in many other organisms. Furthermore, Weksler (1981) has reported that there appears to be an age-associated increase in antinucleoprotein antibody, antithyroglobulin antibody, and rheumatoid factor. In each case there is an increase in autoimmune antibodies with increasing age. One of the most dramatic changes is the nearly fifteenfold increase in rheumatoid factor between the second and ninth decades of life. Similar, but less pronounced, increases were observed in the other two autoantibodies. The presence of the increased percentage of circulating autoantibodies may, in and of itself, not increase health risks in the elderly. However, the presence of autoantibodies increases the possibility that they will combine with antigens to form immune complexes which, in turn, can cause tissue damage. As noted by Weksler (1981), high levels of circulating autoantibodies have been observed in many otherwise healthy elderly people without having the same deleterious pathophysiologic effects that they would have had in the young. At the same time, however, it is possible that the presence of the autoantibodies may produce slowly progressing, low-grade tissue damage to joints, kidneys, and the cardiovascular system. In fact, Walford (1969), in his immunologic theory of aging, has speculated that the cumulative effects of immunologic challenges from foreign antigens as well as from self-antigens produce tissue damage, the accumulation of which can incorrectly be identified as aging.

Of critical importance in this regard is the underlying mechanism responsible for increases in autoantibodies in the elderly. The simplest explanation is that there is a failure of immunologic tolerance with increasing age. That is to say, during development when the immune system first encounters antigens associated with body tissues, a state of immunologic tolerance (immunologic nonresponsiveness) is established so that antibodies to self-antigens (i.e., autoantibodies) are not produced. The failure-of-tolerance explanation holds that as the person or animal ages, tolerance that already exists disappears and antibodies to antigens from normal body tissues are now produced. Although this explanation seems reasonable, there is no published evidence that provides direct support for it. Rather, research has shown that tolerance *induction* becomes more difficult with increasing age. For example, Dobken, Weksler, and Siskind (1980) have reported that it is more difficult to induce B-cell tolerance in old NZB mice, a strain that normally exhibits high levels of autoantibodies as they age, than in the young from that strain when dinitrophenol was used as the immunogen. Furthermore, when young, thymectomized, irradiated syngeneic mice were reconstituted with B cells from the spleens of young animals, tolerance induction was normal for the age group. However, when similar treated young animals were reconstituted with B cells from the spleens of old donors, tolerance induction was not complete. Consistent with these findings are results which show that there is a decrease in high affinity clones of B cells from older animals (Dobken et al., 1980). It is possible that B cells from aged donors have a reduced ability to become tolerant to self-antigens because they are of the low affinity phenotype and bind poorly with self-antigens, making it more difficult to produce tolerance.

Whatever the reason for the increased difficulty to *induce* tolerance in old animals, it is important to realize that the ease or difficulty of tolerance induction in the old mouse is not a direct measure of the failure of tolerance with increasing age (i.e., the explanation given for the increased levels of autoantibodies in aged mice). In short, the failure of tolerance is not equivalent to age-related increases in the ability to induce tolerance. Furthermore, it is possible that the increased autoantibody levels that are seen in aged animals and humans arise not because of a failure of tolerance. Rather, they could occur as a result of the emergence of neoantigens or as a result of antigens that had been suppressed during early development, but are expressed during old age. Thus the increase in autoantibodes may merely reflect the normal response of the immune system to "new" antigens that it does not recognize and hence to which it is responsive. The results of the study cited by Weksler (1981) suggest that it would be more difficult for old subjects to become tolerant to neoantigens, thus increasing the chances for the occurrence of pathological conditions resulting from immune complexes of autoantibodies and the new self-antigens. Unfortunately, there is no direct evidence regarding the occurrence of neoantigens or the emergence of suppressed antigens in aged animals or humans, so this explanation remains entirely speculative. Moreover, as we will see subsequently, it is possible that the increase in autoantibodies could simply result from age-related perturbations in regulation of antibody-producing cells.

Overall, then, the humoral immune response, like the cellular immune response, appears to be impaired with advancing age. The degree of impairment, however, appears to be much less than that which exists in the cellular immune response. The effects of the impairment may, however, be no less important. In fact, as explained in the next section, it is possible that much of what is seen as a defect in the humoral response of aged subjects may not be intrinsic to B cells. These age-related changes may, instead, reflect concomitant aging changes in the regulatory functions of other parts of the immune system.

It has been suggested that many of the aging changes in various physiological systems can best be understood in terms of changes in the ability of the aged organism to maintain homeostasis or a steady state in response to changes in environmental events. Most students of the aging organism agree that with increasing age it becomes more difficult for the organism to maintain a homeostatic state. Indeed, one noted gerontologist has used the term "homeostenosis" to refer to the changes that characterize the aged organism's ability to adapt to environmental change.

The immune system appears to be no exception insofar as regulatory functions are concerned. A recent report by Astle and Harrison (1984) illustrates the overall nature of the regulatory changes that occur in the immune system of aged organisms. In this study, lethal irradiation followed by the transplantation of bone marrow and thymuses from young mice restored both T- and B-cell response in old mice. When mice receive 650 to 750 R of whole body radiation, there is total destruction of all functional immune cells and their precursors. It is possible to reconstitute immune function by transplanting bone marrow from genetically compatible donors. In the Astle and Harrison study, transplants of bone marrow from either young or old donors restored these immune responses in young mice, whereas bone marrow transplants from old mice to old mice did not. So far these findings are generally consistent with those already reported in other similar studies. However, Astle and Harrison went one step further in attempting to understand why the marrow cells from old mice were not effective in reconstituting the immune response in other old mice but were effective in young mice. They parabiosed pairs of mice by surgically connecting their peritoneal cavities in order to allow lymphocytes from the two animals to commingle. Results showed that old mice parabiosed to a young partner and young mice parabiosed to an old partner produced significantly lower immunoresponsivess (relative to young mice parabiosed to a young partner) in both the B- and the T-cell compartments. One interpretation of these findings is that there is a suppressive factor contained in the bone marrow of old mice that is expressed in the environment of an old immune system, but not in that of a young one. As we shall see, the documented age-related changes in immunoregulation are consistent with this interpretation in that, overall, there appears to be a down-regulation or shift to a suppression-dominated control of the aging immune system. However, before detailing the specific age-related changes in regulation that occur, let us examine some of the elements involved in immunoregulation.

Evidence leading to the conclusion that T cells are involved in regulatory processes comes from at least two sources. On the one hand, it has been observed that neonatally thymectomized mice do not develop the ability to reject skin grafts from other mice. In retrospect, this result is not surprising since it was known that, without a functional thymus, T cells could not mature and produce a population of T cells necessary for the graft-rejection reaction. More striking, however, is the finding that neonatally thymectomized mice also developed no response or, at best, a poor *humoral* immune response to sheep red blood cell antigens as well as to foreign serum proteins. Both cellular and humoral responses could, however, be restored by thymus grafts from a compatible donor, suggesting that the cellular and humoral components of the immune system interact.

A second line of evidence comes from studies involving the restoration of immune function in lethally irradiated mice. In early experiments, however, it was observed that mice which had been thymectomized and irradiated recovered the function of *both* cellular and humoral immunity only if they received thymic transplants along with bone marrow reconstitution. Thus it appeared that the cellular arm of the immune system, or some part of it, was cooperating with the humoral immune response. It took subsequent experiments, including those that identified distinctive phenotypic subsets of T cells that served distinctive regulatory functions, to establish that T-helper cells enhanced and/or made possible humoral immunoresponsiveness to certain types of anitgens, while T-suppressor cells interfered with or dampened antibody responses.

It should be noted at this point that not all antibody responses are under T-cell-dependent regulatory control. Whether or not an antibody response is T-dependent or T-independent depends on the nature of the antigenic challenge. T-dependent antigens are, for the most part, proteins while T-independent antigens include many carbohydrates as well as the lipopolysaccharides of certain bacteria. There are other characteristics of T-independent antigens which distinguish them from T-dependent antigens. For example, T-independent antigens, referred to as polyclonal activators, stimulate B cells to differentiate into antibody-secreting cells—even B cells that do not have the specific receptors for the antigen. Also, most T-independent antigens stimulate IgM antibodies which, in turn, exhibit poor immunologic memory.

The effects of aging on *T-dependent* regulation of immune responses can best be seen in the results of a cell transfer experiment (Weksler, Innes, & Goldstein, 1978). In this experiment young mice were lethally irradiated and thymecto-mized. They were then reconstituted with T and B cells from donors of different ages. Immune responses to antigenic challenge were found to be dependent on the age of the donor of the T cells. If these cells came from old donors, the antibody response was reduced and was characterized by low-affinity antibodies (i.e., those that combined poorly with antigen). If, on the other hand, T cells came from young donors, the antibody responses were not impaired. Further analysis showed that the defect appeared to be localized with the T-helper subset obtained from the old donors. These cells appeared to be only one-third to one-tenth as active as those taken from young animals. That the B-cell deficit in old mice is dependent on T-cell factors was further confirmed in this study. Lymphocytes from old animals were transferred to irradiated animals with intact thymuses. If the old animals had been treated with thymic hormones before cells were taken or if the lymphocytes were incubated in thymic hormone prior to transfer, B-cell response to antigen was augmented. If not, B-cell response was comparable to that of an old animal.

There are several possible explanations for the regulatory changes that occur with advancing age. On the one hand, it is known that T-cell development is retarded in old mice by the decreased capacity of these animals to produce and bind interleukin-2 (IL-2), a hormone-like substance, to T cells (Gillis, Kozak, Durante, & Weksler, 1981). Thus the fact that levels of IL-2 are reduced in older animals and the fact that the IL-2 which is produced binds poorly to developing cells in old animals provides a more than adequate basis for the retarded development of regulatory T cells, such as the T-helper subset. Furthermore, Miller (1984) has reported a three- to five-fold decline in the precursors of helper T cells in old animals. Corresponding to the decline in precursors, Miller also reported a reduction in IL-2 which also transforms precursors to natural killer cells (i.e., "resting" cells) into functional lymphocytes. Natural killer cells are T cells that are thought to be involved in host defense reactions against tumors and viruses. Miller's results are particularly important because they indicate that, *on a per cell basis*, the amount of IL-2 produced by old animals is not different from the amount produced by young ones. However, it appears that fewer cells in old animals than in young ones become activated and subsequently secrete IL-2. In passing it should be noted that this is not an isolated finding. Several investigators have reported that other types of cells from aged animals, once activated, are as capable of producing an effect as are cells from young animals. The difference between young and old appears to be that fewer cells from old donors become activated and hence the total effect appears to be diminished in these animals.

That IL-2 is important in restoring the antibody response in old animals was demonstrated in a study reported by Thoman and Weigle (1981). They showed that the ability of spleen cells from old animals to produce antibodies in a plaque assay was enhanced by the addition of IL-2 to the cells. More recently they have shown that the addition of IL-2 to cultures of spleen cells also restores the regulatory function of T-suppressor cells taken from old mice (Thoman & Weigle, 1983). It should not be concluded from these findings, however, that the age-related deficit in the production of antibodies is caused solely by deficits in the T-helper/suppressor cell compartment of the immune system or by deficits in IL-2 production. It has been suggested that there may also be other deficits in the interaction between T and B cells as well as in the B cells themselves. It is known, for example, that certain T-cell functions (e.g., antigen-specific prolif-eration) can be completely restored by the addition of IL-2 to cell cultures from old animals. At the same time, however, IL-2 only partially restores in vitro B-cell function. The difference in the restorative effects of IL-2 on these two cell types is suggestive of another, non-lymphokine, defect in B cells from old mice. One such possibility is that B cells from old mice are less responsive to the modulating factors produced by T cells, even when these factors are produced by T cells from young mice. To date there are no data that directly address this possibility. However, recent evidence reported by Klinman (1981) shows that, while the size of the population of B cells does not change appreciably with increasing age, the expressed specificity (i.e., the specific antigen binding sites) and perhaps other stimulating factors do appear to decline, *on a per cell basis*. In other words, it is possible that fewer B cells are responsive to regulatory control in old than in young animals.

There is yet another regulatory network that appears to change with age and which may have an impact on age-related changes in B-cell function. This network is referred to as the idiotype network. An idiotype is an antigen com-bining site on a particular antibody that is unique for that antibody and distin-guishes it from other antibodies. A "lock-and-key" analogy is often used to describe the distinctive relationship between the antigen molecules and the idi-otype of the receptor molecule on the cell. Regulation that occurs via the idiotype network involves the action of internally produced antibodies to the idiotype (i.e., referred to as auto-anti-idiotypic antibodies or simply as auto-anti-ids). The idiotypic network is responsive to both T-dependent and T-independent antigens. For example, when a T-independent antigen, such as trinitrophenol (TNP)-Ficoll, is introduced into a cell culture, there is proliferaton of B cells that express receptors of a TNP-Ficoll idiotype. Mature B lymphocytes with this idiotype differentiate and proliferate into antibody-secreting plasma cells that are also characterized by the idiotype for the TNP-Ficoll antigen. Once the antibody recognizes and eliminates the antigen, the idiotype stimulates the production of a second set of B cells which, in cooperation with T-helper cells, produce anti-idiotypic antibody-producing plasma cells. Once the anti-idiotypic antibodies reach a critical level they exert a suppressive effect on the idiotype of the original antibody-secreting B cell, presumably through the action of a subset of T-suppressor cells, causing a cessation of the immune response.

Extensive research on the aging changes involved in this regulatory network has been conducted by Goidl and his colleagues. Basically they have reported (e.g., Goidl, Thorbecke, Weksler, & Siskind, 1980) an increase in the production of anti-idiotypic antibody in a TNP-Ficoll-stimulated system using cells from aged mice. They have also found that idiotype expression appears to be age specific. That is to say, the idiotypes expressed on B cells from young animals were different from those expressed on the cells from old animals. If we think of an idiotype as the "lock" part of the "lock-and-key" arrangement of antigen and antibody, then age-related changes in the "lock" without concomitant changes in the "key" can produce significant regulatory changes such as a dampening or down-regulation of the immune response.

Age-related increases in auto-anti-ids have also been reported using a T-dependent antigen system (Szewczuk & Campbell, 1980). Moreover, increased auto-anti-id production can be transferred to lethally irradiated young recipients by transplanting spleen cells but not bone marrow cells from old donors (Goidl et al., 1983). This suggests that the aging changes in the production of auto-anti-ids are intrinsic to the peripheral B cells and not to the bone marrow cells. In other words, the defect does not occur until the B cells enter peripheral circulation, perhaps when they interact with regulatory T cells.

It appears, then, that whether or not we focus on the T-cell aspects or on the idiotypic network apects of regulation, there is a tendency for the aged immune system to be suppressed or down-regulated in its responsiveness to foreign antigens. It has been noted by several investigators (e.g., Goidl, in press; Weksler, 1981) that this dampening effect on the entire system may, in fact, be an adaptive response of the aged immune system to suppress age-associated increases in autoantibodies. According to this argument, without such a down-regulation, an accumulation of autoantibody-antigen complex with the potential of causing extensive physical damage to various tissues and organs could occur. In other words, many of the changes in B-cell function noted in the previous section could be the inadvertent consequence of an adaptive age-related change in immunoregulation.

Thus far we have focused on changes in regulation at the level of the lymphocyte. There are, however, other age-related changes that can be traced to the biochemical level. On the one hand, it is known that the hormones of the adrenal-pituitary axis, namely the corticosteroids, are immunosuppressive. Fauci, Dale, and Balow (1976), for example, administered 400 mg of hydrocortisone to a normal volunteer and then measured circulating T and B cells at 2, 4, 6, 8 and 24 hours after the injection. Results showed that by 4 hours the total number of lymphocytes had decreased by one-fourth (T cells were 75% below baseline while B cells were approximately 66% below baseline). Independent studies that will be reviewed in detail in a subsequent section of this chapter have shown that, following the administration of a stressor, basal levels of plasma corticosterone are elevated in old rats and that these levels remain high for a longer period of time than in young rats. It is possible that age-related changes in hormonal status, similar to those observed with corticosterone, could induce powerful regulatory changes in immune functioning in the elderly. For example, it is possible that a particular stressor could have greater immunosuppressive effects in an aged individual than in a young one. However, to date little or no research has addressed questions like this.

Another biochemical system that has powerful regulatory control over immune function involves the cyclic nucleotide or second messenger system. The cyclic nucleotides, cyclic AMP (cAMP) and cyclic GMP (cGMP), are known as second messengers in that they transmit signals from outside of the cell (e.g., from hormones) to the nucleus of the cell. Levels of these two biochemicals are known to be important to lymphocyte differentiation and proliferation (Klimpel, Byers, Russell, & Lucas, 1979; Watson, 1975). Walford and his colleagues (e.g., Tam & Walford, 1981) have reported striking changes with increasing age in cAMP and cGMP levels in splenic T cells of mice as well as in T cells from peripheral blood in humans. There is, for example, a nine- to tenfold increase in cGMP in older humans with a corresponding twenty-fivefold increase in cAMP. According to early notions about levels of these two biochemicals, increases in the ratio of cAMP to cGMP leads to decreases in cell proliferation and increases in cell differentiation. Thus it is consistent with these notions that lymphocytes from old animals and humans, in which there is an age-associated increase in the cAMP-cGMP ratio, proliferate poorly but differentiate at an accellerated rate. It was noted earlier that, in old individuals, there is a large population of mature or differentiated T cells but these cells appear to respond (i.e., to proliferate) poorly to mitogens.

Finally, aged lymphocytes appear to be defective at the most elemental, the genetic, level of regulation. At the present time the data are meager because research is just beginning in this area. However, many investigators have reported that lymphocytes from aged individuals are deficient in the ability to repair damage to DNA, the basic structure responsible for cell proliferation (Lambert, Ringbord, & Swanbert, 1977; Seshadri, Morley, Trainor, & Sorrell, 1979). Also, it was noted earlier that Staiano-Coico et al. (1983) found that lymphocytes from aged humans are more susceptible to genetic damage and cell-cycle arrest caused by the low levels of tritiated thymidine used in the standard assays of proliferative capacity of lymphocytes.

In summary, it appears that, at every level of analysis, there are major defects in the regulation of the immune system of aged individuals. Most of these regulatory changes can explain many of the specific phenomena that have been documented from the study of aged immune systems. Indeed, one could argue that the primary age-related change in immune function is in immunoregulation and that other observed changes derive from these regulatory changes. Moreover, it appears that the nature of these regulatory changes is to down-regulate or dampen immunoresponsiveness. Thus the aged immune system appears to be able to make normal responses to mitogens and antigens, but it makes them less vigorously than does the young immune system.

NUTRITIONAL FACTORS IN THE AGING IMMUNE SYSTEM

Research using a variety of approaches has consistently shown that nutritional factors play an important role in either forestalling or overcoming many of the age-related changes in immune functioning that have been outlined in previous sections. The topic of nutritional factors in immune functioning has received considerable attention elsewhere (e.g., Fernandez, 1984; Schneider & Reed, 1986; Weindruch, 1984) and, therefore, only a few highlights will be presented here. The reader is encouraged to refer to these excellent reviews.

In aging research the topic of most active interest has been the effects of dietary restriction on immune function. This work stems from the early observation published by McCay, Crowell, and Maynard (1935) that rats raised on a food-restricted diet without malnutrition had longer mean and maximal life spans than those raised on "normal" laboratory diets. Subsequent research has focused on the specific dietary constituent(s) that could have produced this effect. One hypothesis is that caloric restriction in some way maintains maximal immune function throughout the life span of the animal, thus minimizing the life-shortening effects of disease (e.g., from infectious agents or tumors). Indeed, research has shown that caloric restriction initiated either at weaning or at midlife enhances B- and T-cell function to various antigens and mitogens (Weindruch, Gottesman, & Walford, 1982). Further, it has been found that restriction of certain dietary constituents (e.g., fat content) also enhances many aspects of immune function and forestalls the onset of autoimmune disease in strains of mice that are highly susceptible to it. The interleukins and prostaglandins appear to be particularly affected by restriction of dietary fat content (Fernandez, 1984). However, to date it is not known how the restriction of fat content affects these particular aspects of immune function.

Many of the studies on dietary restriction have limited caloric intake without paying attention to the specific constituents that are restricted or eliminated from the diet. It is known, though, that certain nutrients are needed for normal immune function and that supplementation with these nutrients can ameliorate age-induced changes in immune function (e.g., see Fernandez, 1984). The trace metal zinc, for example, is necessary for normal development of thymic tissue and related T-cell function. In addition, animals deficient in zinc exhibit depressed plaque-forming responses to sheep red blood cells and depressed natural killer cell activity. Thus, although caloric restriction can forestall loss of immune function in aged animals, if certain key nutrients are omitted from the diets of developing animals, interference with normal immune function can occur.

At this stage in the development of research on dietary restriction there are many issues that still need to be resolved. One involves the method used to retrict the diet. For example, is it sufficient to feed animals ad lib on alternate days in order to restrict the dict by 50%? Research from the behavioral sciences would suggest that, since animals appear to adapt their feeding patterns to the scheduled availability of food in order to maintain their caloric intake at a *relatively* constant level, alternate day feeding may not be an adequate method to *reduce* caloric intake. Related to this is the observation that restricted animals are more active than ad lib-fed animals. This raises the question whether or not the same effect on immune function could be produced by exercising the animals without limiting intake. If the same effect could be produced, to what extent is the dietary restriction per se (vs. the exercise) responsible for the effects of restriction on immune function? Moreover, are the effects produced by exercise alone mediated by the same physiological/biochemical mechanism(s) as those produced by diet alone? Another question concerns the nature of the mechanism that underlies the effects of dietary manipulations. Is there a direct biochemical effect on cells and tissues of the immune system (e.g., those affecting cell membrane motility) or could these effects occur as a result of indirect influences of dietary manipulations on other systems (e.g., via the endocrine system or CNS)? Finally, it is reasonable to ask whether or not the effect has anything to do with caloric restriction per se. It has been noted that animals receiving a restricted diet are also ingesting a smaller amount of "toxins" that might be present in the food. Thus, dietary restriction might reduce the challenge to the developing immune system and, in so doing, prolong its effectiveness in later life. In summary, at present we know that dietary restriction has important immunorestorative effects on the aging immune system. We do not, however, know how or why these effects occur. Many of the questions that need to be answered are the kinds that have been dealt with by biobehavioral scientists. Thus, it appears that significant contributions can be made by the behavioral sciences.

PSYCHONEUROENDOCRINE INFLUENCES
ON THE AGING IMMUNE SYSTEM

One question that arises naturally from a study of the aging immune system concerns the extent to which age-related changes in immune function occur as a result of aging changes that are inherent to the components of the immune system (e.g., those resulting from aging changes in tissue or cellular physiology) as opposed to those that result from concomitant aging changes in systems that interact with the immune system (e.g., in the CNS or endocrine system). From this perspective, one can ask questions about the degree to which aging changes in T-cell proliferation, for example, are caused by changes in thymic physiology as opposed to aging changes in the broader hormonal milieu of T cells (e.g., the levels of corticosterone, calcium-regulating, or growth hormones; the receptors for various hormones; the action of the hormones across cell membranes; etc.). In addition, it is also reasonable to ask about the degree to which aging changes in immune functioning influences what have been identified as age-related changes in other systems.

Thus far we have focused primarily on the aging changes that take place within the immune system, although earlier mention was made of the fact that there appear to be extensive interconnections among the CNS, the endocrine system, and the immune system. In the present section, we will consider briefly the impact of some aging changes in other systems on immune functioning and vice versa. At the outset it is important to note that the purpose of the present section is not to review what is becoming an extensive body of literature on the interaction between the immune system and other homeostatic systems of the body. This has already been done, most notably in the comprehensive book entitled *Psychoneuroimmunology* by Robert Ader (1981). Instead, what I intend to do here is to review research that appears to be leading in a direction that may help to uncover answers to questions about potential interrelationships among aging changes in the CNS, the endocrine system, and the immune system.

One approach to studying these interrelations is exemplified in a study by Sapolsky and Donnelly (personal communication, 1984) involving the interaction between aging changes in corticosterone levels and tumor growth in male rats. Prior studies had uncovered the finding that the adrenal cortex is relatively insensitive to negative feedback from products of the pituitary-adrenal cortex axis in aged male Fischer 344 rats (e.g., Sapolsky, Krey, & McEwen, 1983a; Sapolsky, Krey, & McEwen, 1983b; Landfield, Waymire, & Lynch, 1978; DeKosky, Scheff, & Cotman, 1980). This loss of negative feedback appears to result from a reduction in glucocorticoid receptors in brain regions that mediate negative feedback signals. As a consequence, aged rats exhibit higher basal levels of corticosterone (11 ug/100 ml) than do young rats (6 mg/100 ml) and, following exposure to a stressor, levels of corticosterone return to basal levels more slowly in the aged rats. A corticosterone profile similar to that observed in old animals was also reported to have been found in young rats if they received a 100 mg injection of corticosterone at the end of one hour of restraint stress.

Sapolsky and Donnelly extended these observations by examining the impact of stress on tumor rejection and growth in young and old animals. In this experiment both age groups were injected with a premeasured dose of Fischer fetal rat cells that had been transformed with Fujinami sarcoma viruses. The dose of cells used had, in a previous study, been determined to be below the threshold for producing measurable tumor growth in the young animals within a one-month time period. Experimental animals were then subjected to one of eight different stressors every three hours for seven days. Controls were returned to their home cages and remained undisturbed during this period. Two weeks after the stress sessions ended the animals were sacrificed and tumor number and size were measured. Results showed that there were no differences in the number of tumors observed among the four groups. Tumor size, as measued by weight, however, differed greatly among the groups. Both stressed and non-stressed young animals had tumors averaging less than 100 mg, as did the older non-stressed animals. However, the average size of tumors in the old stressed rats was approximately 1250 mg, a difference which was reliably greater than the other three groups. Findings similar to those obtained in the old stressed rats were reported for young animals that had received a 100 mg injection of cor-ticosterone following each stressor. However, in this case, two weeks after the end of the stress sessions the tumors were somewhat smaller than those observed in the old stressed subjects (i.e., approximately 900 mg). It was not until three weeks post-stress that average tumor size in these young, stressed, injected animals reached the size observed two weeks post-stress in the old stressed animals.

These findings suggest that age-related changes in an endocrine function can, under the proper conditions, have an influence on the rate of tumor growth. It is important to realize, however, that they do not necessarily indicate that age-related changes in endocrine function have a direct, or even an indirect, influence on *immune function* per se—even though such a conclusion is tempting. This conclusion cannot be drawn because no direct measurements of immune func-tioning were made in this study and because it is known that glucocorticoids can affect the rate of tumor growth via pathways other than the immune system (e.g., by influencing cell metabolic processes). At the same time, however, the role of immune factors cannot be ruled out entirely since it is also known that tumor size can be influenced by a variety of immunologic factors, most of which, in turn, are affected by glucocorticoids. Thus these data provide an important and promising foundation upon which future investigations into the influence of age-related changes in hormonal status on various aspects of immune function can be based.

A second example of research that stresses the interactive aspects of immune functioning involves a study by Kiecolt-Glaser and her colleagues on the amelioration of stress-induced changes in immunoresponsiveness in a geriatric population. In a series of early studies, not involving a geriatric population, they showed that natural killer cell activity was lower in medical students at the time of final exams than it had been when they returned from summer vacation (Kiecolt-Glaser et al., 1984a; Kiecolt-Glaser, Speicher, Holliday, & Glaser, 1984b). Kiecolt-Glaser et al. (1984a, 1984b) also observed that, at both times, subjects scoring above the median on a measure of loneliness had reliably lower natural killer cell activity than did subjects below the median. Analysis of immunocompetence showed that antibodies to each of three herpesviruses [Epstein-Barr virus, herpes simplex virus Type I (HSV-I) and cytomegalovirus] were elevated at exam time compared to samples taken at the time of return from summer vacation (Glaser, et al, 1985).

The notion underlying this research is that the stress associated with exams or loneliness compromises certain aspects of immune functioning, namely that aspect which controls the onset of viral infection. It is thought that after an active herpesvirus infection, the viruses remain within the cells that they have infected but their action is repressed by the cellular arm of the immune system. However, when an individual is immunosuppressed (for example, at a time of stress such as during exams), the latent viruses are reactivated, causing an increase in virus-produced antigen. As with any antigenic challenge, an increase in antibodies specific to the particular herpesvirus antigenic determinant occurs in order to counteract the presence of the antigens. Thus, the increase in antibody level in this particular system is taken as an indirect measure of immunosuppression of the cellular arm of the immune system, as well as a direct measure of the action of the humoral arm of the immune system against the herpesvirus antigen.

Kiecolt-Glaser and her colleagues (Kiecolt-Glaser et al., 1985) have extended their analysis of stress effects on immunocompetence to a geriatric population. They approached the problem by arguing that the heightened levels of infectious disease observed in nursing home populations may, in no small way, result from loneliness- and/or stress-induced immunosuppression in the residents. Also, they noted that other research has shown that nursing home residents appear to be responsive, both psychologically and physiologically, to interventions designed to reduce both loneliness and stress (e.g., Rodin, 1980; Schulz, 1980). Therefore, they designed an intervention study to examine the relationship between stress/loneliness reduction on immunocompetence in nursing home residents.

Subjects, ranging in age from 60 to 88 years, were selected from four independent living facilities. They were ambulatory, capable of caring for their own personal needs, able to communicate verbally, and had no identified medical problems involving an immunologic component or leading to immunologic consequences. Residents were assigned to one of three treatment groups which received: (1) relaxation training three times a week for one month, (2) social contact control via visits from college students three times a week for one month, and (3) no contact following the initial interview. Blood samples were taken from individuals in all three groups for immunologic assays prior to the beginning of intervention (baseline), one month later (at the end of the intervention period), and one month after the end of intervention. Three kinds of immunologic assays were obtained from each blood sample: (1) a chromium release measure of the cytotoxicity of natural killer cells, (2) the enzyme-linked immunosorbent assay of antibody activity to HSV-I, and (3) responsiveness of cells to pokeweed mitogen, which stimulates both T and B cells to proliferate, and to PHA, which stimulates only T cells to proliferate.

Results showed that relaxation training was effective in enhancing natural killer cell cytotoxicity and in lowering HSV-I antibody levels. These changes, for the most part, were maintained at the follow-up assessment one month after the intervention ceased. No other groups showed reliable changes in these two measures of immunoresponsiveness, nor did any of the measures of proliferative capacity of T and B cells reflect the differential effect of any of the treatments. Thus it appears that relaxation training (the alleviation of stress?) can have palliative effects on some immune functions related to the health of nursing home elderly.

Two additional aspects of these studies are worth examining. It should be noted at the outset that the statistical comparisons upon which these conclusions are based were not made by Kiecolt-Glaser et al. in any of their published data, and therefore they are speculative in nature. Any errors in generalization are, thus, the responsibility of the present author and not those of Kiecolt-Glaser et al. The first observation is that, overall, the levels of proliferation, at each concentration of mitogen, appeared to be lower at baseline in the geriatric population than in the younger medical students used in the previous studies. These age differences in proliferative capacity are consistent with other published studies and indicate that the elderly population used by Kiecolt-Glaser et al. was probably not atypical of the geriatric population as a whole. Secondly, similar age-related differences can be detected when the natural killer cell cytotoxicity data are compared between the nursing home residents and the medical students. As far as the present author can determine, this is the first published indication that natural killer cell cytotoxiciy may, along with proliferative capacity, deline with advancing age. What is particularly interesting is that the mean level of cytotoxicity of natural killer cells from the elderly who received relaxation training was nearly identical, numerically, to that obtained from cells taken from the medical students following summer vacation. These comparisons suggest that the relaxation method used for the elderly in this study was sufficiently powerful to increase certain aspects of immune function to a level comparable to that of young, and presumably healthy, individuals.

The preceeding two research examples show that extra-immunologic factors (i.e., endocrine and psychological) can have an important and dramatic impact on the functioning of the aging immune system. It is also possible for age-related changes in immune function to have an impact on other physiologic systems.

For example, it was noted in a previous section of this chapter that there is an age-related increase in the level of brain-reactive autoantibodies (BRA). These BRAs appear to increase with age in mice, rats, nonhuman primates and man (e.g., Nandy, 1972a, 1981a, 1981b; Chaffee, Nassef, & Stephen, 1978). Nandy (1975) has shown that BRAs react specifically with brain tissue, as well as with cells around the blood-brain barrier (Nandy, 1972b, 1975), although slight cross-reactivity with thymic tissue has also been noted. These autoantibodies appear to be of the gamma-globulin class and are not necessarily produced by stimulation from extrinsic pathogens as was shown in a study in which age-related increases in BRA occurred in mice raised under typical laboratory conditions as well as in those raised under germ-free conditions (Nandy, 1972b). In a more recent study, Nandy and Bennett (1983) examined the role of the aging immune system in the formation of BRA. In this study they demonstrated that it was possible to adoptively transfer BRA from old mice to young, irradiated, syngeneic animals. Specifically, they transplanted bone marrow cells to young mice who, at the age of 5–6 months, developed levels of BRA comparable to those observed in control mice 20–24 months of age. Since 5-month-old mice do not typically exhibit the presence of any BRAs, the increases observed in this study were not only statistically significant, but they were also biologically important. In addition, neither mature T or B cells appeared to be necessary for this effect to occur, nor did the addition of suppressor cells to the transplanted bone marrow cells suppress the accumulation of BRA in either young or old recipients. Further, when stem cells from young mice were transferred to old irradiated recipients, BRA levels in the hosts remained high, suggesting that the young animals did not possess a transferable suppressor factor that was controlling the expression of BRA. However, when old animals were thymectomized and then injected with bone marrow cells along with a thymus graft from young donors, there was a statistically reliable decline in BRA in the old recipients. Thus, it appears that the age-related increase in BRA is related, in some way, to the age-related decline in thymic functioning. The specific aspect of thymic function that underlies this effect is still to be determined but may be related to the well-documented age-related decline in thymic hormone level.

Research on BRA not only is important for a fuller understanding of the aging immune system, but it also may be important to gaining a fuller understanding of the the etiology of certain diseases of the elderly. It has been suggested, for example, that senile dementia may result from the destructive action that BRA has on cells of the CNS. It would be informative to document the specific age-related behavioral changes that parallel the action of BRA. In this regard, it would also be instructive to map, in detail, the sites and progresssion of action of BRA in the CNS. Finally, it would also be informative to know whether or not dementia that is caused by experimental administration of BRA (e.g., as in the Nandy and Bennett study) produces behavioral changes that are equivalent to those that may occur in untreated aging animals. In short, it is clear that there are many opportunities for additional research in this area and that the behavioral sciences can make important contributions.

Again, I want to stress the fact that examples cited above have been selected because they point to new and important areas of research involving the aging immune system. The first example focuses on the impact of age-related changes in endocrine function on immunoresponsiveness. This kind of research can be extended to (a) cover many hormones in addition to the glucocorticoids (e.g., calcitonin, parathyroid hormone, estrogen, etc.), (b) address questions about the mechanisms that cause aging changes (e.g., receptor changes, changes in the "potency" of the hormonal product, etc., and (c) other systems (e.g., CNS). Similarly, the work by Kiecolt-Glaser et al. points to another approach that can produce important information about the aging immune system. Specifically, I am referring to the fact that their work points to potential methods for ameliorating the age-related decline in immune function and the concomitant increase in immunogenic diseases. Their work also points to the potential of future research aimed at examining the way in which age-related changes in immune function can influence aging changes in other systems. Finally, the studies on BRA can further our understanding of one of the most costly and devastating diseases of the elderly, senile dementia. If nothing else, it may also help us to understand the ways in which autoantibodies can produce age-related changes in other systems which, in turn, may ultimately have an impact on immune functioning. Consider, for example, the possibility that age-related increases in BRA to cells involved in the regulation of a hormone such as corticosterone could modify the function of those cells in such a way that subsequent corticosterone levels would be increased as in the study by Sapolsky and Donnelly. As a consequence, it is possible that the immunogenic changes in endocrinologic function could cause additional immunologic changes that appear to be age-related. Obviously, speculation like this is not very useful without experimental verification. It does, however, point to the potential pervasiveness of rather small age-related changes in the immune system in the organism as a whole and, therefore, may be useful in stimulating and organizing future research.

CONCLUSION

In reviewing what is known about the aging immune system, it becomes immediately apparent that most of our knowledge focuses on the adaptive responses of the system to antigenic challenges, while little is known about the aging changes that involve the role of the immune system in the larger homeostatic network. This is not entirely surprising since research on the immune system, in general, has tended not to address this issue, and little is known about the interaction of immune function with other systems or the mechanisms involved in this interaction. Interestingly, however, the study of the aging immune system in and of itself or in relation to other parts of the homeostatic network may provide leadership in the field of psychoneuroimmunology by helping us to understand the interactive relationships among the various components. Thus, research on the impact of age-related changes in hormonal systems (e.g., glucocorticoids) on various aspects of immune function (e.g., lymphocyte proliferation) may provide not only an understanding of the causes of age-related changes in immune function, but also clues about the general role of immune-endocrine interactions in the maintenance of homeostasis.

Behavioral research on the aging immune system has been sparse and has focused on the impact of what might be termed sociobehavioral or life stresses on immune capacity. While this research is certainly important and can lead to useful findings regarding health problems in the elderly, it is also important for the behavioral sciences to begin to expand this research. For example, research aimed at assessing the influence of aging changes in immune capacity on social networks, personality, or other behavioral variables can provide important insight into the pervasive influences of the aging immune system as well as offer yet another potential physiological basis for understanding behavioral changes in aging. Similarly, further development of research on the impact of age-related changes in behavior on immune function is needed. However, it is particularly important in this kind of research that investigators select immunologic variables that are biologically meaningful to the aging process and/or aged individuals. The reason for this is that, generally speaking, behavioral scientists currently involved in research in this area are interested in discovering the connections between behavioral events and the state of the individual's health. The assumption underlying this approach, which is often referred to as behavioral medicine, is that the effect of behavior on health is mediated by behaviorally induced physiologic processes. In the present instance, these physiologic responses involve the immune system. In attempting to uncover the interrelationships of behavior, immune function, and health, many behavioral scientists have relied primarily on suppression of T-cell proliferation as a measure of total immunoresponsiveness. The research by Kiecolt-Glaser et al., however, shows that some measures of immunoresponsiveness may be affected by a given behavioral manipulation (i.e., relaxation training), while other measures may not. Further, their work also points to the importance of selecting measures of immune function that are related to the individual's health. T-cell proliferative responses to a mitogen may reflect immune processes that are only indirectly involved in a given disease process, while another measure of immune function (e.g., the production of an antibody to a specific antigenic determinant) may represent a more direct assessment of health status. The latter measure, then, should be the dependent variable of choice in this kind of research.

In addition, it is important in research of this type for investigators to show that there is, in fact, at least correlative evidence between changes in immune function and health status. Thus, even though an investigator provides evidence for behaviorally induced immunosuppression or immunorestoration, it is important to show also that there were concomitant predictable changes in the health status of the experimental subjects. An experiment reported by Ader and Cohen (1982) serves as a prototype of the kind of experiment to which I am referring. In this experiment it was found that not only could immunosuppression in NZB × NZW mice be conditioned but also that the conditioning created a change that ameliorated the age-dependent onset of systemic lupus erythematosus. This change was reflected both in the physiologic measuresused to assess the progression of the disease and in the survival rates of animals in various treatment and control groups. The important point here is that, without confirming evidence that behavioral manipulations influence both physiologic and health variables, the connections between behavior, immune function, and health will remain speculative. Finally, it is important to note that because of the highly specialized nature of immunologic assays and methods, to say nothing about the esoteric nature of the data base of the field itself, behavioral scientists should be prepared to become involved in truly interdisciplinary research.

The emphasis on behavioral issues in the foregoing paragraphs should not be taken to mean that research on aging changes in the various comonents of the immune system itself is not important. In fact, our current knowledge of age-related changes in immune functioning points to some very important and fruitful areas for future research. In particular, it is important for us to continue to focus on the mechanisms underlying the regulatory changes in the aging immune system. Information about membrane and internal lymphocyte events undoubtedly will provide important clues about age-related changes in regulatory function. Similarly, much additional research is required before we will have a full understanding of the mechanisms underlying aging changes in intracellular communication via the interleukins, hormones, and idiotypic antibodies. Further, additional information is needed about the role of various genetic influences on aging changes in immune capacity.

Finally, a major research effort is needed on certain important clinically relevant issues. We need to understand the mechanisms that underlie the immunorestorative effects of techniques such as dietary restriction and/or relaxation training. Furthermore, there is still much to be learned about the immunologic basis of infectious diseases in the elderly, including the effectiveness of various vaccines in preventing infections. In summary, while we have learned much about the aging immune system in the past 20 years or so, there is still much more to be discovered.

REFERENCES

Ader, R. A. (Ed.). (1981). *Psychoneuroimmunology*. New York: Academic Press.

Ader, R. A., & Cohen, N. (1982). Behaviorally conditioned immunosuppression and murine systemic lupus erythematosus. *Science, 215*, 1534–1536.

Arrenbrecht, S., & Sorkin, E. (1973). Growth hormone-induced T cell differentiation. *European Journal of Immunology, 3*, 601–604.

Astle, C. M., & Harrison, D. E. (1984). Effects of marrow donor and recipient age on immune responses. *Journal of Immunology, 132*, 673–677.

Bach, J. F., Dardene, M., Pleu, J. M., & Bach, M. A. (1975). Isolation, biochemical characteristics and biological activity of circulating thymic hormone in the mouse and in the human. *Annals of the New York Academy of Science, 249*, 186–210.

Bach, M. (1979). Influence of aging on T cell subpopulations involved in the in vitro generation of allogeneic cytotoxicity. *Clinical Immunology and Immunopathology, 13*, 220–230.

Besedovsky, H., & Sorkin, D. (1977). Network of immune-neuroendocrine interactions. *Clinical Experimental Immunology, 27*, 1–12.

Blistein-Wellinger, E., & Deinenstein, T. (1978). Inhibition by isoptin (a calcium antagonist) of mitogenic stimulation of lymphocytes prior to the S-phase. *Immunology, 34*, 303–307.

Boyd, E. (1932). The weight of the thymus gland in health and in discase. *American Journal of Diseases in Children, 43*, 1162–1214.

Bulloch, K., & Moore, R. Y. (1980). Innervation of the thymus gland by brain stem and spinal cord in mouse and rat. *American Journal of Anatomy, 162*, 157–166.

Chaffee, J., Nassef, M., & Stephen, R. (1978). Cytotoxic antibody to the brain. In K. Nancy (Ed.), *Senile dementia: A biomedical approach* (pp. 61–72). New York: Elsevier.

Chapman, M. L., Zaun, M. R., & Gracy, R. W. (1981). Effects of age on energy status of redox state of lymphocytes during blastogenesis. *Biochemistry and Biophysics Research Communications, 98*, 303–310.

DeKosky, S., Scheff, S., & Cotman, C. (1980). Elevated corticosterone levels: A possible cause of reduced axon sprouting in aged animals. *Neuroendocrinology, 38*, 33–38.

Dobken, J., Weksler, M. E., & Siskind, G. W. (1980). Effect of age on B-cell tolerance induction. *Cellular Immunology, 55*, 66–73.

Fauci, A. S., Dale, D. C., & Balow, J. E. (1976). Glucocorticosteroid therapy: Mechanisms of action and clinical considerations. *Annals of Internal Medicine, 84*, 304–321.

Fernandez, G. (1984). Nutritional factors: Modulating effects on immune function and aging. *Pharmacology Reviews, 36*, 123–129.

Friedman, D., & Globerson, A. (1978). Immune reactivity during aging. II. Analysis of the cellular mechanisms involved in the deficient antibody response in old mice. *Mechanisms of Aging Development, 7*, 299–307.

Friedman, D., Keiser, V., & Globerson, A. (1974). Reactivation of immunocompetence in spleen cells of aged mice. *Nature, 25*, 545–547.

Gillis, S. C., Kozak, R., Durante, M., & Weksler, M. E. (1981). Immunlogic studies of aging: Decreased production of and response to T cell growthh factor by lymphocytes from aged humans. *Journal of Clinical Investigation, 67*, 937–942.

Glaser, R., Kiecolt-Glaser, J. K., Speicher, C. E., & Holliday, J. E. (1985). Stress, loneliness and changes in herpesvirus latency. *Journal of Behavioral Medicine, 8*, 249–260.

Goidl, E. A. (In Press). Aging and autoimmunity. In E. D. Goidl (Ed.), Aging and the immune responses. New York: Marcel Decker.

Goidl, E. A., Choy, J. W., Gibbons, J. J. Weksler, M. E., Thorbecke, G. J., & Siskind, G. W. (1983). Production of auto-anti-idiotypic antibody during the normal immune response. VII. Analysis of the cellular basis for the increased auto-anti-idiotypic antibody production by aged mice. *Journal of Experimental Medicine, 157*, 1635–1645.

Goidl, E. A., Thorbecke, G. J., Weksler, M. E., & Siskind, G. W. (1980). Production of auto-anti-idiotypic antibody during the normal immune response: Changes in the auto-anti-idiotypic antibody response and the idiotypic repetoire with aging. *Proceedings of the National Academy of Sciences, 77*, 6788–6792.

Goldstein, A. L., & Zatz, M. (1981). Thymosin and aging. In D. Segre & L. Smith (Eds.), *Immunological aspects of aging* (pp. 371–390). New York: Marcel Dekker.

Goldstein, G. (1975). The isolation of thymopoietin (thymin). *Annals of the New York Academy of Sciences, 249*, 177–185.

Hall, N. R. S., McGillis, J. P., & Goldstein, A. G. (1984). Activation of neuroendocrine pathways by thymosin pathways. In E. Cooper (Ed.), *Stress, immunity and aging* (pp. 209–224). New York: Marcel Dekker.

Hallgren, H. M., Buckley, C. E., Gilbertson, V. A., & Yunis, E. J. (1973). Lymphocyte phytohemagglutinin responsiveness, immunoglobulins and autoantibodies in aging humans. *Journal of Immunology, 111*, 1101–1107.

Hefton, J. M., Darlington, G. J., & Casazza, B. A. (1980). Immunologic studies of aging. V. Impaired proliferation of PHA responsive human lymphocytes in culture. *Journal of Immunology, 125*, 1007–1110.

Hirokawa, K., & Makinodan, T. (1975). Thymic involution: Effect on T cell differentiation. *Journal of Immunology, 114*, 1659–1664.

Inkeles, B., Innes, J. B., & Kuntz, M. M. (1977). Immunological studies of aging. III. Cytokinetic basis for impaired response of lymphocytes from aged humans to plant lectins. *J. Exp. Med., 145*, 1176–1187.

Joncourt, F., Kristensen, F., & deWeck, A. L. (1982). Age-related changes in g0-g1 transition and proliferative capacity of mitogen-stimulated murine spleen cells. *Gerontology, 28*, 281–289.

Kennes, B., Hubert, C., & Broher, D. (1981). Early biochemical events associated with lymphocyte activation in aging. I. Evidence that Ca2 + dependent processes induced by PHA are impaired. *Immunology, 1*, 119–126.

Khachaturian, A. K. (1984). Towards theories of brain aging. In D. W. K. Kay & G. D. Burrows (Eds.), *Handbook of studies on psychiatry and old age* (pp. 7–30). New York: Elsevier.

Kiecolt-Glaser, J. K., Garner, W., Speicher, C., Penn, G. M., Holliday, J., & Glaser, R. (1984a). Psychosocial modifiers of immunocompetence in medical students. *Psychosomatic Medicine, 46*, 7–14.

Kiecolt-Glaser, J. K., Speicher, C. E., Holliday, J. E., & Glaser, R. (1984b). Stress and the transformation of lymphocytes by Epstein-Barr virus. *Journal of Behavioral Medicine, 7*, 1–12.

Kiecolt-Glaser, J. K., Glaser, R., Welliger, D., Stout, J., Messick, G., Sheppard, S., Bnnnell, G., & Dnnnenberg, R. (1985c). Psychosocial enhancement of immunocompetence in a geriatric population. *Health Psychology, 4*, 25–41.

Klimpel, G. R., Byers, C. V., Russell, D. H., & Lucas, D. O. (1979). Cyclic AMP-dependent protein kinase activation and the induction of ornithine decarboxylase during lymphocyte mitogenesis. *Journal of Immunology, 123*, 817–824.

Klinman, N. (1981). Antibody-specific immunoregulation and the immunodeficiency of aging. *Journal of Experimental Medicine, 154*, 547–551.

Lahita, R. G. (1982). Sex hormones and immunity. In D. P. Stites, J. D. Stobo, H. H. Fudenberg, & J. V. Wells (Eds.), *Basic and clinical immunology* (4th ed., pp. 293–297). Los Altos, CA: Lange Medical Publications.

Lambert, B., Ringbord, N., & Swanbert, B. (1977). Repair of UV-induced DNA lesions in peripheral lymphocytes from healthy subjects of various ages, individuals with Down's syndrome and patients with actinic peratosis. *Mutation Research, 46*, 133–134.

Landfield, P. W., Waymire, J. C., & Lynch, G. (1978). Hippocampal aging and adrenocorticoids: Quantitative correlations. *Science, 202*.

Linten-Moore, S. (1977). Effect of athymia on the initiation of follicular growth in the rat ovary. *Biological Reproduction, 17*, 155–161.

Makinodan, T., & Adler, W. H. (1975). The effects of aging on the differentiation and proliferation of potentials of cells of the immune system. *Federation Proceedings, 34*, 153–158.

Makinodan, T., & Kay, M. M. B. (1980). Age influence on the immune system. *Advances in Immunology, 29*, 287–330.

McCay, C. M., Crowell, M. F., & Maynard, L. A. (1935). The effects of retarded growth upon the length of life span and upon ultimate body size. *Journal of Nutrition, 10*, 63–79.

Miller, R. A. (1984). Age-associated decline in precursor frequency for different T cell-mediated reactions, with preservation of helper or cytotoxic effect per precursor cell. *Journal of Immunology, 132,* 63–68.

Miller, R. A., & Stuttman, O. (1981). Decline in aging mice of the anti-2,4,6-trinitrophenyl (TNP) cytotoxic T cell response attributable to loss of Lyt2-, interleukin 2-producing helper cell function. *European Journal of Immunology, 11,* 751–756.

Moody, C. E., Innes, J. B. Staiano-Coico, L., Incefy, G. S., Thaler, H. T., & Weksler, M. E. (1981). Lymphocyte transformation induced by autologous cells. XI. The effect of age on the autologous mixed lymphocyte reaction. *Immunology, 44,* 431–438.

Nandy, K. (1972a). Brain-reactive antibodies in mouse serum as a function of age. *Journal of Gerontology, 24,* 173–177.

Nandy, K. (1972b). Brain-reactive antibodies in germ-free mice. *Mechanisms of Aging Development, 1,* 133–138.

Nandy, K. (1972c). Neuronal degeneration in aging and after experimental degeneration. *Experimental Gerontology, 7,* 303–311.

Nandy, K. (1975). Significance of brain-reactive antibodies in serum of aged mice. *Journal of Gerontology, 30,* 412–416.

Nandy, K. (1981a). Brain-reactive antibodies in aging non-human primates. *Mechanisms of Aging Development, 16,* 141–146.

Nandy, K. (1981b). Senile dementia: A possible immune hypothesis. In J. A. Mortimer & M. Shuman (Eds.), *Epidemiology of senile dementia* (pp. 87–100). New York: Oxford University Press.

Nandy, K., & Bennett, M. (1983). Immune manipulations and brain-reactive antibody formation in aging mice. *Mechanisms of Aging Development, 22,* 287–293.

Patel, P. J. (1981). Aging and antimicrobial immunity: Impaired production of mediator T cells as a basis for the decreased resistance of senescent mice to lysteriosis. *Journal of Experimental Medicine, 1981, 154,* 821–831.

Paul, J. R., & Bunnell, W. W. (1952). Anti-SRBC agglutinin with age. *American Journal of Medical Sciences, 183,* 90–97.

Pierpaoli, W., & Besedovsky, H. O. (1975). Role of the thymus in programming of neuroendocrine functions. *Clinical Experimental Immunology, 20,* 323–328.

Rebar, R. W., Mijake, A., Low, T. L., & Goldstein, A. L. (1981). Thymosin stimulates secretion of luteinizing hormone-releasing factor. *Science, 214,* 669–671.

Roberts-Thompson, I. C., Whittinghaus, S., & Youngchaiyud, U. (1974). Aging, immune response and mortality. *Lancet, 2,* 368–370.

Rodin, J. (1980). Managing the stress of aging: The role of control and coping. In S. Levine & H. Ursin (Eds.), *Coping and health* (pp. 171–202). New York: Plenum.

Rosenberg, J. S., Gilman, S. C., & Feldman, J. D. (1982). Activation of rat B lymphocytes. II. Functional and structural changes in 'aged' rat B lymphocytes. *Journal of Immunology, 128,* 656–660.

Sapolsky, R. M., Krey, L. C., & McEwen, B. S. (1983a). The adrenocortical stress response in the aged male rat: Impairment of recovery from stress. *Experimental Gerontology, 18,* 55–64.

Sapolsky, R. M., Krey, L. C., & McEwen, B. S. (1983b). Corticosterone receptors decline in a site-specific manner in the aged rat brain. *Brain Research, 289,* 235–240.

Schneider, E. L., & Reed, J. D. (1985). Modulations of aging processes. In C. E. Finch & E. L. Schneider (Eds.), *Handbook of the biology of aging* (2nd ed., pp. 45–76). New York: Van Nostrand Reinhold.

Schulz, R. (1980). Aging and control. In J. Garber & M. E. P. Seligman (Eds.), *Human helplessness: Theory and applications* (pp. 261–277). New York: Academic Press.

Segre, D., & Segre, M. (1976). Humoral immunity in aged mice. II. Increased suppressor T cell activity in immunologically deficient old mice. *Journal of Immunology, 116,* 735–738.

Seshadri, R. S., Morley, A. A., Trainor, K. J., & Sorrell, J. (1979). Sensitivity of human lymphocytes to bleomycin increases with age. *Experimentia, 35*, 233–234.

Singh, J., & Singh, A. K. (1979). Age-related changes in human thymus. *Clinical Experimental Immunology, 37*, 507–511.

Staiano-Coico, L., Darzynkewicz, Z., Hefton, J. M., Dutkowski, R., Darlington, G. J., & Weksler, M. E. (1983). Increased sensitivity of lymphocytes from people over 65 to cell cycle arrest and chromosomal damage. *Science, 219*, 1335–1337.

Stuttman, O. (1981). Thymic hormones, T cell development and aging. In D. Segre & L. Smith (Eds.), *Immunological aspects of aging* (pp. 333–370). New York: Marcel Dekker.

Szewczuk, M. R., & Campbell, R. J. (1980). Loss of immune competence with age may be due to auto-anti-idiotypic antibody regulation. *Nature, 286*, 164–166.

Talal, N., Dauphinee, M. J., & Roubinien, J. R. (1981). The effect of sex hormones and thymosin on autoimmunity. In d. Segre & L. Smith (Eds.), *Immunological aspects of aging* (pp. 415–421). New York: Marcel Dekker.

Tam, C. F., & Walford, R. L. (1981). Alterations in cyclic nucleotides and cyclase-specific activities in T-lymphocytes of aging normal humans and patients with Down's syndrome. *Journal of Immunology, 125*, 1665–1670.

Thoman, M., & Weigle, W. (1981). Lymphokines and aging: Interleukin 2 production and activity in aged animals. *Journal of Immunology, 127*, 2102–2106.

Thoman, M., & Weigle, W. (1983). Deficiency in suppressor T cell activity in aged animals: Reconstitution of this activity by interleukin 2. *Journal of Experimental Medicine, 157*, 2184–2189.

Tranin, N., Small, M., Zipori, D., Umiel, T., Kook, A. I., & Rotter, V. (1975). Characteristics of THF, a thymic hormone. In D. W. VanBekkum (Ed.), *The biological activity of thymic hormones* (pp. 117–144). Rotterdam: Kooyker Scientific Publication.

Verity, M. A., Tam, C. F., Cheung, M. K., Mock, D. C., & Walford, R. L. (1983). Delayed phytohemagglutinin-stimulated production of adenosine triphosphate by aged human lymphocytes: Possible relation to mitochondrial dysfunction. *Mechanisms of Aging Development, 23*, 53–65.

Waldorf, D. S., Wilkens, R. R., & Decker, J. L. (1968). Impaired delayed hypersensitivity in an aging population: Association with antinuclear reactivity and rheumatoid factor. *Journal of the American Medical Association, 203*, 831–834.

Walford, R. L. (1969). *The immunologic theory of aging*. Baltimore: Williams and Wilkins.

Watson, J. (1975). The influence of intracellular levels of cyclic nucleotides on cell proliferation and the induction of antibody synthesis. *Journal of Experimental Medicine, 141*, 91–111.

Weindruch, R. H. (1984). Dietary restriction and the aging process. In D. Armstrong, R. Sohal, R. Cutler, & T. F. Slater (Eds.), *Free radicals in molecular biology, aging, and disease* (pp. 181–202). New York: Raven Press.

Weindruch, R. H., Gottesman, S. R. S., & Walford, R. L. (1982). Modulation of age-related immune decline in mice dietarily restricted from or after mid-adulthood. *Proceedings of the National Academy of Sciences, 79*, 898/902.

Weindruch, R. H, Krisite, J. A., Naeim, F., Mullen, B. G., & Walford, R. L. (1982). Influence of weaning-initiated dietary restriction on response to T cell mitogens and on splenic T cell levels in a long-lived F1-hybrid mouse strain. *Experimental Gerontology, 17*, 49–64.

Weksler, M. E. (1981). The senescence of the immune system. *Hospital Practice, 16*, 53–64.

Weksler, M. E., Innes, J. B., & Goldstein, G. (1978). Immunological studies of aging. IV. The contribution of thymic involution to the immune deficiencies of aging mice and reversal with thymopoietin 32–36. *Journal of Experimental Medicine, 148*, 996–1006.

Williams, J. M., Peterson, R. G., Shea, P. A., Schmedtje, J. F., Bauer, D. C., & Felten, D. C. (1981). Sympathetic innervation of murine thymus and spleen: Evidence for a functional link between the nervous and immune systems. *Brain Research Bulletin, 6*, 83–94.

Woda, B. A., & Feldman, J. D. (1979). Density of surface immunoglobulin and capping on rat B lymphocytes. I. Changes with aging. *Journal of Experimental Medicine, 149*, 416–423.

8

IMMUNITY AND AGING
Experimental and Clinical Studies

Marvin Stein
Steven J. Schleifer
Steven E. Keller
Mount Sinai School of Medicine
of the City University of New York

A range of biopsychosocial factors has been considered in relation to an organism's response to stressful and other environmental stimuli. It has been suggested by Riley that aging must also be taken into account and attention be directed to the interaction of biological and psychosocial processes as they influence one another from birth to death (Riley, in press). The immune system is one of the major integrative networks involved in biological adaptation. Considerable evidence demonstrates that a variety of psychosocial factors influences the central nervous system (CNS) which thereby may result in the suppression or enhancement of immune function. This chapter will review experimental and clinical studies concerned with the influence of stress and other psychosocial processes on immunity as well as consider some of the psychobiological mechanisms which may be involved. The research was not designed specifically to investigate the influence of aging, however a time perspective is implicit. The studies will not be presented in Riley's time frame of aging from birth to death but, rather, will be described following a time sequence from death to birth.

THE IMMUNE RESPONSE

Before considering specific aspects of psychosocial effects on immune function, it is important to have a general understanding of the various components of the immune system. The immune response is responsible for the maintenance of the integrity of the organism in relation to foreign substances such as bacteria, viruses, tissue grafts, and neoplasia.

The immune system can be divided into two major aspects: cell-mediated and humoral immunity. The basic cellular unit of both cell-mediated and humoral immunity is the lymphocyte, however the lymphocytes in each immune component are different. The T lymphocyte is primarily involved in cell-mediated immunity, and the B lymphocyte is involved in humoral immunity. Both T and B lymphocytes derive from pluripotent stem cells in the bone marrow with T-cell maturation in the thymus. Several subsets of T cells have been described and include helper-T cells, suppressor-T cells and effector-T cells. In addition to T and B lymphocytes, a number of other cell types are involved in immune processes and include monocytes, macrophages, mast cells, and neutrophils.

In the development of an immunologic response, antigens, substances recognized as foreign, attach to lymphocytes genetically programmed to recognize a specific antigen. When antigens bind to the surface of lymphocytes, division of the cells occurs, resulting in lymphocyte proliferation and effector responses. Upon reexposure to the antigen, a more rapid and extensive secondary response occurs due to the induction of memory developed in a subset of lymphocytes during the proliferative component of the primary response.

In humoral immunity, sensitized B lymphocytes, following activation by signals from macrophages and T-helper cells, proliferate and differentiate into plasma cells which synthesize antigen-specific antibodies. The primary protective function of humoral immunity is against infections by encapsulated bacteria (e.g., streptococci). At times, however, the response can be pathological, as in anaphylaxis, asthma, and, occasionally, in response to the organism's own tissues in an autoimmune disorder such as systemic lupus erythematosus.

In contrast to the B cell whose role is primarily secretory, the T cell itself participates in the cell-mediated immune response. Genetically controlled T lymphocytes passing through the tissues are sensitized to a specific antigen peripherally and progress to a local lymph node where they enter the free areas of the cortex follicles. The T cells proliferate and are transformed into larger lymphoblasts. After several days, the T lymphocytes become immunologically active. One subpopulation of effector-T lymphocytes mediates delayed-type hypersensitivity such as occurs in chemical-contact sensitivity or in the tuberculin reaction. Another subpopulation of T cells are cytotoxic or, upon contact with the antigen, release lymphokines such as macrophage migration inhibitory factor (MIF), chemotactic factors, cytotoxic factors, and interferon. The lymphokines are involved in the destruction of the antigen. Cell-mediated immune responses include protection against viral, fungal, and intracellular bacterial infection; transplantation reactions; and immune surveillance against neoplasia.

The classical division of the immune system into cellular and humoral immunity is oversimplified. Recent research has revealed that the immune system consists of highly fine-tuned and self-regulatory processes with T to T and T to

B lymphocyte interdependence and interactions. These regulatory functions may have both protective and pathological effects on the organism.

Many studies have used lymphocyte stimulation as an in vitro correlate of cellular immunity. Lymphocyte stimulation is an in vitro technique which is commonly used to assess the in vivo function and interaction of lymphocytes involved in the immune response. In the procedure, sensitized lymphocytes are cultured and activated with specific antigens, or non-sensitized cells are activated with nonspecific stimulants known as mitogens. A number of plant lectins and other substances have been used as mitogens. Phytohemagglutinin (PHA) and concanavalin A (ConA) are predominantly T-cell mitogens, and pokeweed mitogen (PWM) stimulates primarily B lymphocytes.

When lymphocytes are stimulated, there is an increase in DNA synthesis, which eventually results in cell division and proliferation. The measurement of DNA synthesis is made by labeling stimulated cultures with a radioactive nucleoside precursor which is incorporated into newly synthesized DNA. The determination of the amount of precursor incorporated provides a measure of DNA synthesis and is employed as the standard measure of lymphocyte responsiveness. The radioactive incorporation data are expressed as counts per minute (CPM), and the CPM in unstimulated cultures is substracted from the stimulated CPM and provides a stimulation index (ΔCPM).

BEREAVEMENT, DEPRESSION, AND LYMPHOCYTE FUNCTION

Conjugal breavement is among the most potentially stressful of commonly occurring life events and has been associated with increased medical mortality. Helsing, Szklo, and Comstock (1981), in a prospective study of mortality after widowhood, found that in males between the ages 55 and 74, the relative risk of mortality was significantly greater in the widowed group than in a group of married matched controls. No difference in mortality rates were found comparing widowed and married women.

We have investigated the effect of bereavement on immunity in a prospective longitudinal study of spouses of women with advanced breast carcinoma (Schleifer, Keller, Camerino, Thornton, & Stein, 1983). Twenty spouses of women undergoing treatment for advanced metastatic disease in the Department of Neoplastic Diseases, Mount Sinai Hospital, New York, were studied. Spouses were entered into the study during a three-year period, and each subject was studied at approximately six- to eight-week intervals for the duration of the patient's illness. Lymphocyte measures were obtained for 15 of these subjects during the first two months following the death of spouse. Twelve of the 15 were also studied during the four- to fourteen-month post-bereavement period. On entry into the study, the subjects had a mean age of 57 years and had been married

30 years; the spouse's diagnosis had been made an average of 2.5 years prior to entry. Subjects were observed for a mean of six months from entry into the study to death of spouse.

The mitogen-induced lymphocyte stimulation responses, measured in the 15 men before and after the death of their wives, are shown in Figure 8.1. The responses to the mitogens PHA, ConA, and PWM were significantly lower during the first two months after bereavement compared with pre-bereavement responses. The number of peripheral blood lymphocytes and the percentage and absolute number of T and B cells obtained during the pre-bereavement period were not significantly different from those obtained during the post-bereavement period. Follow-up during the remainder of the post-bereavement year revealed that lymphocyte stimulation responses had returned to pre-bereavement levels for the majority but not all of the subjects. Moreover, pre-bereavement mitogen responses did not differ from those of age- and sex-matched controls. These findings demonstrate that suppression of mitogen-induced lymphocyte stimulation is a direct consequence of the bereavement event, and that a preexisting suppressed immune state does not account for the depressed lymphocyte response in the bereaved. Furthermore, the long-term stress of the spouse's illness does not appear to result in a habituation of lymphocyte stress responses following bereavement. The long term stress may, in fact, have sensitized the subjects (Burchfield, 1979) to the effects of bereavement.

The effects of bereavement on lymphocyte function in our sample, however, were not homogeneous. A small subset of subjects did not have lowered mitogen responses at 1–2 months post-bereavement but tended to have decreased levels when restudied during the latter half of the post-bereavement year. It is of note that these subjects were younger than the majority of the sample who had lowered responses immediately following the death of spouse and a return to pre-bereavement levels after a number of months. Futher systematic investigation of this variability in post-bereavement immune changes is required, including consideration of age, biological predisposition, personality, and changes in life style and behavior associated with bereavement. Furthermore, it is important to emphasize that the immune findings associated with bereavement do not adequately explain the epidemiologic findings of increased morbidity and mortality following bereavement. It remains to be determined whether stress-induced immune changes such as decreased mitogen responses are related to the onset or course of physical illnesses following life stress (Schleifer, Keller, & Stein, 1984).

The processes linking the experience of bereavement with effects on lymphocyte activity are complex and remain to be determined. Changes in nutrition, activity, and exercise levels (Bistrian, Blackburn, & Serimshaw, 1975), sleep (Clayton, 1979), and drug use (Baker, Santalo, & Blumenstein, 1977; Sherman, Smith, & Middleton, 1973; Tennenbaum, Ruppert, & M. St. Pierre), which are often found in the widowed (Clayton, 1979) could influence lymphocyte function.

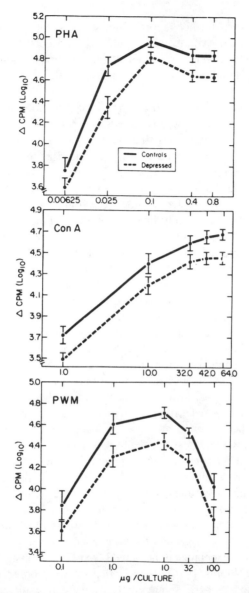

FIGURE 8.1. PHA-, ConA-, and PWM-induced lymphocyte stimulation before and after (one to two months) bereavement. Each point represents group mean ± SEM ($n = 15$) of each subject's mean log change in counts per minute (CPM) for each period. Adapted from "Suppression of lymphocyte stimulation following bereavement" by S. J. Schleifer, S. E. Keller, M. Camerino, J. C. Thornton, and M. Stein, 1983, *Journal of the American Medical Association, 250,* 375. Copyright 1983, American Medical Association.

Our subjects, however, did not report major or persistent changes in diet or activity levels or in the use of medication, alcohol, tobacco, or other drugs, and no significant changes in weight were noted. Further study is required to determine if subtle changes on these variables are related to the effects of bereavement on lymphocyte function.

The effects of death of spouse on lymphocyte function could result from centrally mediated stress effects. Stressful life experiences may be related to changes in CNS activity associated with a psychological state such as depression. Bereaved subjects have been characteristically described as manifesting depressed mood (Clayton, Halikes, & Maurice, 1972; Parkes, 1972), and a subgroup of bereaved individuals has been reported to have symptom patterns consistent with the presence of a major depressive disorder (Clayton et al., 1972).

Immune measures have recently been assessed in clinically depressed individuals. The frequency of antinuclear antibodies, which may reflect autoimmune processes, has been reported to be increased in patients with depression (Deberdt, Van Hooren, Biesbrouck, & Avery, 1976; Shopsin, Sathananthan, Chan, Kravitz, & Gershon, 1973). More recently, investigators have begun to evaluate general measures of lymphocyte function in depression. (Cappel, Gregoire, Thiry, & Sprecher, 1978) reported that lymphocyte stimulation responses to PHA were lower in a group of psychotically depressed patients during the acute phase of their illness than following clinical remission. PHA responses in the depressed group did not differ, however, from those of control subjects at either time, making interpretation of the findings difficult. Kronfol and coworkers (16) reported that melancholic patients had lower lymphocyte responses to PHA, ConA, and PWM than groups of non-melancholic psychiatric patients and normal controls. These studies have been limited by the lack of age- and sex-matched controls being studied on the same day as the depressed patients and by potential interactions between medication effects and lymphocyte function.

We have conducted a series of studies to determine if depressive disorders are associated with altered immunity. Mitogen-induced lymphocyte stimulation and the number of peripheral blood lymphocytes were measured in hospitalized and ambulatory patients with major depressive disorders. Each subject was studied on the same day with an age- and sex-matched apparently healthy control. Depressed subjects were included if they met Research Diagnostic Criteria (RDC; Spitzer, Endicott, & Robins, 1978) for major depressive disorder, had a Hamilton Depression Scale score of 18 or greater (18), were free of acute or chronic medical disorders associated with immune alterations, and were drug free.

In the severely depressed hospitalized patients with major depressive disorder we found evidence of altered immunity (Schleifer et al., 1984). As can be seen in Figure 8.2, lymphocyte stimulation by PHA, ConA, and PWM were significantly lower in the group of hospitalized depressives than in the controls. The total number of T and B cells was also lower in the depressed patients, but the percentage of the cell types did not differ between the groups. These findings

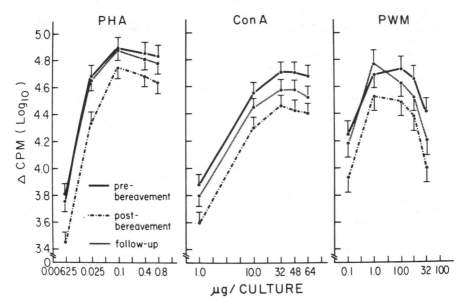

FIGURE 8.2. Mitogen-induced lymphocyte stimulation in hospitalized depressed subjects and controls. Each point represents mean change in counts per minute (ΔCPM) $\pm$ SEM ($n = 18$) log transformed for each group. Adapted from "Lymphocyte function in major depressive disorder" by S. J. Schleifer, S. E. Keller, A. T. Meyerson, M. J. Raskin, K. L. Davis, and M. Stein, 1984, *Archives of General Psychiatry, 41*, 485. Copyright 1985, American Medical Association.

demonstrate that the functional activity of the lymphocyte as well as the number of circulating immunocompetent cells are decreased in individuals hospitalized with acute major depressive disorder.

In order to determine if altered immunity is associated specifically with depression and not related to hospital effects or nonspecifically to other psychiatric disorders, we investigated lymphocyte function in ambulatory patients with major depressive disorder and in patients hospitalized with schizophrenic disorders (Schleifer, Keller, Siris, Davis, & Stein, 1985). Responses to PHA, ConA, and PWM were similar among depressed outpatients and controls (Figure 8.3). The finding of no significant differences in mitogen responses between ambulatory depressives and controls, in contrast to our previous findings of suppressed responses to the same mitogens in hospitalized depressives, suggests that the decreased mitogen responses in the inpatient depressives may be related to hospitalization or to severity of the depression.

A group of hospitalized schizophrenic patients were therefore studied, and we found no differences between the hospitalized schizophrenics and their controls in the response to mitogens (Figure 8.4) nor on any of the quantitative lymphocyte measures. These findings suggest that hospitalization on a psychiatric unit is not in itself sufficient to result in a change in mitogen responsivity or in

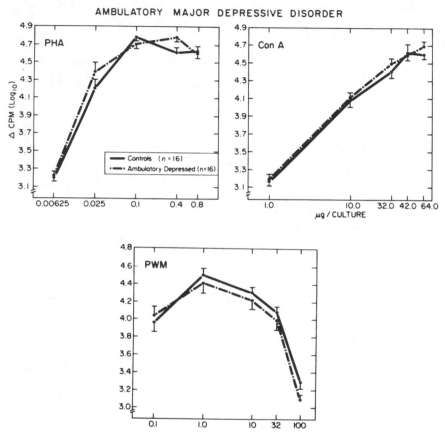

FIGURE 8.3 Mitogen-induced lymphocyte stimulation in ambulatory depressed subjects and controls. Each point represents mean change in counts per minute (ΔCPM) $\pm$ SEM (n = 16) log transformed for each group. From "Depression and immunity. Lymphocyte function in ambulatory depressed, hospitalized schizophrenic, and herniorrhaphy patients" by S. J. Schleifer, S. E. Keller, S. G. Siris, K. L. Davis, and M. Stein, 1985, *Archives of General Psychiatry, 42,* 130. Copyright 1985, American Medical Association.

the number of peripheral blood lymphocytes. It is possible, however, that schizophrenic inpatients are not directly comparable to inpatient depressives since they may have atypical responses to hospitalization. The effect of hospitalization on lymphocyte function was therefore studied in a group of otherwise healthy patients admitted for elective herniorrhaphy, and no significant differences were found between the herniorrhaphy patients and matched controls (Schleifer et al., 1985).

The decreased mitogen responses in hospitalized patients with major depressive disorder but not in ambulatory depressed patients suggest that the altered

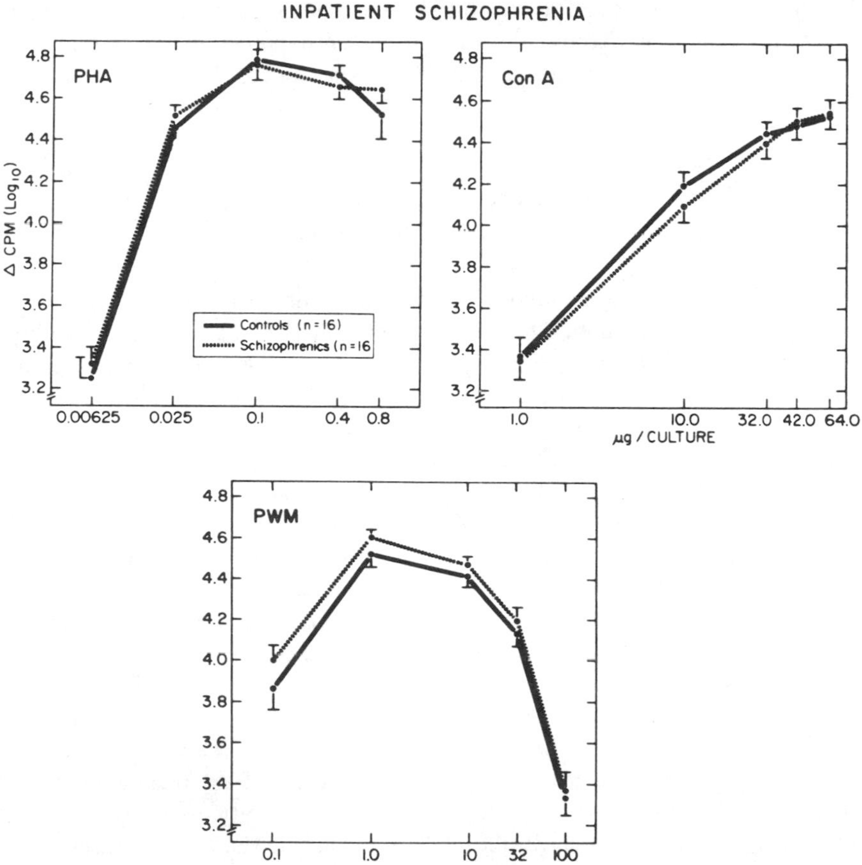

FIGURE 8.4.   Mitogen-induced lymphocyte stimulation in hospitalized schizo-phrenic subjects and controls. Each point represents mean change in counts per minute (ΔCPM) $\pm$ SEM (n = 16) log transformed for each group. From "Depression and immunity. Lymphocyte function in ambulatory depressed, hospitalized schizophrenic, and herniorrhaphy patients" by S. J. Schleifer, S. E. Keller, S. G. Siris, K. L. Davis, and M. Stein, 1985, *Archives of General Psychiatry, 42,* 131. Copyright 1985, American Medical Association.

immunity in depression may be related to severity of depressive symptomatology. The ambulatory patients were less severely depressed by clinical and Hamilton Rating Scale measures as compared to the hospitalized patients. This preliminary observation of an association between altered lymphocyte function and severity of depression suggests that immune changes may be related to underlying bio-logical processes in depression such as a neurotransmitter defect which could be responsible for neuroendocrine dysregulation and immune alterations. Nor-epinephrine, for example, has been shown to have an inhibitory effect on several neuronal subsets in the hypothalamus, and there is evidence that norepinephrine

133

has a tonic inhibitory effect on ACTH and cortisol secretion. A norepine-phrine deficiency in affective disorders has been hypothesized to contribute to the hypercortisolemia associated with depression (Jones, Hillhouse, & Burden, 1976).

MEDIATION OF STRESS EFFECTS
ON IMMUNE FUNCTION

A variety of factors may be involved in mediating the associations among stress, depression, and immunity. The endocrine system is highly responsive to both life experiences and psychological state and has a significant although compli-cated effect on immune processes. The most widely studied hormones are those of the hypothalamic-pituitary-adrenal (HPA) axis. A wide range of stressful experiences are capable of inducing the release of corticosteroids (Coe, Mendoza, Smotherman, & Levine, 1978; Hofer, Wolff, Friedman, & Mason, 1972; Tache, DuRuisseau, Tache, Selyc, & Collu, 1976) and, as noted, cortisol secretion is increased in major depressive disorder. Corticosteroids have extensive and com-plex effects on the immune system. Of particular interest in relation to our findings of decreased numbers of lymphocytes and lower mitogen responses in depression is the demonstration that pharmacological doses of glucocorticoster-oids diminish mitogen-induced lymphocyte stimulation (Fauci, 1975; Fauci & Dale, 1975; Goodwin, Messner, & Williams, 1979) and induce a redistribution of T cells from the circulating pool to the bone marrow (Fauci & Dale, 1975; Claman, 1972). Several reports have demonstrated that the recirculating lym-phocyte traffic in humans is sensitive to endogenous corticosteroids and varies in relation to endogenous cortisol levels (Thomson, McMahon, & Nugent, 1980; Abo, Kawate, Ito, & Kumagai, 1981), as does the response to PHA stimulation (Abo et al., 1981; Tavadia, Fleming, Hume, & Simpson, 1975).

Secretion of corticosteroids has long been considered the mechanism of stress-induced modulation of immunity and related disease processes (Riley, 1981; Selye, 1976). The regulation of immune function in response to stress, however, may not be limited to corticosteroids. We have shown in rats that unpredictable, unavoidable electric tail shock suppressed immune function as measured by the number of circulating lymphocytes and PHA stimulation (Keller et al., 1981). In an effort to determine if the adrenal is required for stress-induced suppression of lymphocyte function in the rat, we investigated the effect of stressors in adrenalectomized animals (Keller, Weiss, Schleifer, Miller, & Stein, 1983). Four groups of rats were studied, consisting of non-operated, adrenalectomized, sham adrenalectomized, and adrenalectomized animals with a corticosterone pellet. The four treatments, home-cage control, apparatus control, low-shock, and high-shock animals, were identical to those used in our previous study. There was a progressive increase in corticosterone with increasing stress in both of the groups with adrenals, no corticosterone was detected in the adrenalectom-ized group, and the concentration of corticosterone in the adrenalectomized group that received the corticosterone pellets was constant. The corticosterone levels in the sham adrenalectomized group indicated that the two-week post-operative period was sufficient to allow recovery to baseline corticosteroid levels and that the operative procedure did not affect stress-related corticosterone responses. The steroid levels in the adrenalectomized group confirm total adrenalectomy. The adrenalectomy-plus-corticosterone-pellet group showed intermediate corti-costerone levels which were nonresponsive to the stress conditions.

In both the non-operated and sham-operated groups, there was a significantly progressive stress-induced lymphopenia. There were no stress-related changes in lymphocyte number in the adrenalectomized or adrenalectomized-with-pellet groups. Lymphopenia following exposure to stress was described as early as 1937 (Harlow & Selye, 1937) and has been associated with adrenal hypertrophy and involution of the thymus and spleen (Marsh & Rasmussen, 1960). It has been shown that stress-induced leukopenia can be prevented by adrenalectomy in mice (Jensen, 1969). The findings of our study demonstrate that stress-induced lymphopenia in the rat occurs in association with stress-induced secretion of corticosteroids and can be prevented by adrenalectomy.

Figure 8.5 shows that the stressful conditions suppressed the stimulation of lymphocytes by PHA in the adrenalectomized animals. The stressors similarly suppressed PHA responses in non-operated animals, replicating our earlier report (Keller et al., 1981), in sham-adrenalectomized rats, and in adrenalectomized animals with steroid replacement. These findings demonstrate that stress-related adrenal secretion of corticosteroids and catecholamines is not required for the stress-induced suppression of lymphocyte stimulation by the T-cell mitogen PHA in the rat. It may well be that there is an adrenal-independent stress-induced depletion of functional subpopulations of T cells or a selective redistribution to lymphoid tissues. A variety of other hormonal and neurosecretory systems may be involved in the adrenal-independent stress-induced modulation of T-cell func-tion. Since corticosteroids have been reported to have differential effects on T- and B-cell populations (Meyer, Meyer, Niehaus, Schlake, & Grundmann, 1980; Roess, Bellone, Ruh, Nadel, & Ruh, 1982), future studies are required to inves-tigate the role of adrenal hormones in stress effects on B-cell functions.

Our findings of adrenal-dependent stress-induced lymphopenia but of adrenal-independent effects on lymphocyte stimulation indicate that stress-induced mod-ulation of immunity is a complex phenomenon involving several, if not multiple, mechanisms. Changes in thyroid hormones, growth hormones, and sex steroids have been associated with exposure to stressors, and all have been reported to modulate immune function (Stein, Keller, & Schleifer, 1981). More recently, an immunoregulatory role has been suggested for a variety of stress-related peptides such as β-endorphin (Gilman, Schwartz, Milner, Bloom, & Feldman, 1982; Shavit, Lewis, Terman, Gale, & Liebeskind, 1984). Furthermore, the

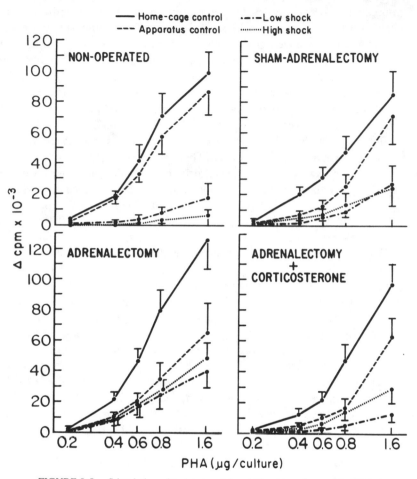

LYMPHOCYTE STIMULATION: Peripheral blood lymphocytes

FIGURE 8.5. Stimulation of isolated peripheral blood lymphocytes by PHA for each of the four operative groups and four treatment procedures. Data (means ± SEM) are presented as ΔCPM (n = 160). From "Stress-induced suppression of immunity in adrenalectomized rats" by S. E. Keller, J. M. Weiss, S. J. Schleifer, N. E. Miller, and M. Stein, September 23, 1983, *Science, 221*, 1302. Copyright 1983 by the American Association for the Advancement of Science.

authors (Keller, Stein, Camerino, Schleifer, & Sherman, 1980; Stein, Schleifer, & Keller, 1982) and others (Cross, Brooks, Roszman, & Markesberry, 1982), have shown that the hypothalamus, which plays a central role in neuroendocrine function, modulates both humoral and cell-mediated immunity. These findings suggest that a range of neuroendocrine processes may be involved in stress-induced altered immunity.

There is good evidence that influences other than hormonal are involved in CNS regulation of immunity. It has been demonstrated in hypophysectomized rats that anterior hypothalamic lesions result in an increase in the number of thymic lymphocytes and a decrease in mitogen response (Cross, Brooks, Roszman, & Markesberry, 1982). A direct link between the CNS and immunocompetent tissues has been suggested by the demonstration of nerve endings in the thymus, spleen, and lymph nodes (Bulloch & Moore, 1980; Calvo, 1968; Giron, Crutcher, & Davis, 1980; Williams et al., 1980). The thymus has also been shown to receive direct innervation from the nucleus ambiguus (Bulloch & Moore, 1980). These findings taken with the presence of adrenergic and cholinergic receptors on the lymphocyte surface (Bourne, Lichtenstein, & Melmon, 1974; Pochet, Delesperse, Gauseet, & Collet, 1979) further support the possibility of a direct link between the CNS and immune response to stressors and in association with psychological states such as depression.

Recently it has been demonstrated that there is decreased norepinephrine turnover in the hypothalamus of the rat at the peak of an immune response, and it has been suggested that the immune response exerts an inhibitory action on central noradrenergic neurons as a result of mediators released by immunological cells (Besedovsky, del Ray, Sorkin, DaPrada, Burri, & Honneger, 1983). Furthermore, it has been shown that the lymphocyte can secrete an ACTH-like substance following viral infection (Smith, Meyer, & Blalock, 1982). These findings suggest the presence of a neuroendocrine-immunoregulatory feedback process associated with aminergic circuits within the CNS.

PREMATURE SEPARATION
AND LYMPHOCYTE FUNCTION

The studies of associations between bereavement and depression and immune function consider the effects of psychosocial processes which occur primarily during the middle and later adult years. Early life experiences, in addition to their immediate effects on biological processes, may induce pervasive long-term effects resulting from the impact of these experiences on psychological and biological systems which are immature and undergoing developmental changes. Premature separation of an infant from its mother is a behavioral intervention which has been shown to alter both CNS and endocrine function and, in humans and animals, can have both immediate and long-term effects on behavior and health (Hofer, 1981). There are an increasing number of studies concerned with early life separation experiences and immune function. Prematurely separated rat pups have decreased resistance to implanted Walker sarcoma (Friedman, Glasgow, & Ader, 1969), and prematurely separated mice have been shown to have an impairment of humorally mediated immune responses (Michaut et al., 1981). We have investigated the effect of premature weaning on lymphocyte stimulation by PHA measured in the adult rat (Keller et al., 1983).

Premature separation was associated with a significant lymphopenia and the response of peripheral blood lymphocytes to PHA was significantly lower in the prematurely separated rats than in normal weaned animals. There was a trend for the response to be lower in males. Consistent with previous studies (Ackerman, Hofer, & Weiner, 1977), both male and female prematurely separated animals weighed less than normally weaned animals.

These findings demonstrate that premature separation of rat pups from their mothers at 15 days of age is associated, at 40 days, with lymphopenia and decreased functional responses of peripheral blood lymphocytes to T-cell mitogen stimulation. The mechanisms underlying the effects of premature separation on peripheral blood lymphocytes require elucidation. The lower weights in the prematurely weaned rats are consistent with a possible nutritional role.

Previous studies have shown that a variety of processes regulated by the hypothalamus are modified by premature maternal separation. It has been demonstrated that premature separation produces alterations in temperature, sleep, metabolic rate and the maturation of autonomic processes (Hofer, 1981; Ackerman, Hofer, & Weiner, 1979). As previously noted, we have demonstrated that lesions in the hypothalamus in mature guinea pigs can suppress both humoral and cell-mediated immune processes, including lymphocyte stimulation responses to PHA (Stein et al., 1981). The effects of premature separation on the immune system may therefore be mediated by altered hypothalamic function (e.g., hypothalamic-pituitary-adrenal axis).

The effects of premature separation on the numbers of peripheral blood lymphocytes and on PHA responsivity directly parallel the changes we have found in adult rats exposed acutely to electric tail shock (Keller et al., 1981). Similar mechanisms may contribute to the effects of tail shock and premature separation on immunity despite the behavioral divergence of the two paradigms.

It remains to be determined if the effects of premature separation on immune function result from a persistent alteration in immunoregulatory systems such as in neuroendocrine function or if the premature separation induces a permanent change in the immune system due to disruption of the normal maturation of the immune system at an important developmental stage. Schanberg and coworkers, for example, found that separation of rat pups from their mothers at 14 days resulted in a rapid decrease in the levels of both ornithine decarboxylase (Butler, Suskind, & Schanberg, 1978), a critical enzyme in protein biosynthesis, and growth hormone (Kuhn, Butler, & Schanberg, 1978), which is required for the normal development of the immune system (Denckla, 1978).

In order to determine the persistence of the deficits in lymphocyte responsivity in prematurely separated rats, we intended to study a second group of rats at 100 days of age. One half of the animals were prematurely separated, and all of the rats were then to be left undisturbed in their cages until 100 days. However, prior to the test age, a large number of these animals developed symptoms of severe respiratory infection and were destroyed by the animal caretaker according to standard laboratory policy. Upon review, all of the diseased animals were found to have been prematurely separated. Segregated housing does not explain these findings since all animals were housed together, with early and normal weaned animals paired in the cage racks. Several diseased rats were autopsied and pneumonitis was apparent but no pathogens could be cultured. These observations suggest a need for further studies to determine if the decrease in lymphocyte stimulation responses found at 40 days is an index of illness susceptibility.

SUMMARY

Considerable evidence demonstrating a relationship between immune function and stress, depression, and other psychosocial processes is accumulating and an extensive network of CNS and neuroendocrine processes may be involved. Further consideration must be given to the role of aging in relation to homeostatic mechanisms involved in the neuromodulation of immune function. Changes in integrative processes associated with aging may result in the modification of adaptive responses to environmental stressful stimuli.

ACKNOWLEDGMENT

This research was supported in part by project grants MH37774 and MH39651 from the National Institute of Mental Health and by the Chernow Foundation.

REFERENCES

Abo, T., Kawate, T., Ito, K., & Kumagai, K. (1981). Studies on the bioperiodicity of the immune response. 1. Circadian rhythms of human T, B, and K cell traffic in the peripheral blood. *Journal of Immunology, 126,* 1360–1363.

Ackerman, S. H., Hofer, M. A., & Weiner, H. (1977). Some effects of a split litter cross foster design applied to 15-day-old pups. *Physiological Behavior, 19,* 433–436.

Ackerman, S. H., Hofer, M. A., & Weiner, H. (1979). Sleep and temperature regulation during restraint stress in rats is affected by prior maternal separation. *Psychosomatic Medicine, 41,* 311–319.

Baker, G. A., Santalo, R., & Blumenstein, J. (1977). Effect of psychotropic agents upon the blastogenic response of human T-lymphocytes. *Biological Psychiatry, 12,* 159–169.

Besedovsky, J., del Ray, A., Sorkin, E., DaPrada, M., Burri, R., & Honegger, C. (1983). The immune response evokes changes in brain noradrenergic neurons. *Science, 221,* 564–566.

Bistrian, B. R., Blackburn, G. L., & Serimshaw, N. S. (1975). Cellular immunity in semistarved states in hospitalized adults. *American Journal of Psychiatry, 28,* 1148–1155.

Bourne, H. R., Lichtenstein, L. M., & Melmon, K. L. (1974). Modulation of inflammation and immunity by cyclic AMP. *Science, 184,* 9–28.

Bulloch, K., & Moore, R. Y. (1980). Nucleus ambiguus projections to the thymus gland. *Abstracts of the American Association of Anatomy,* 25A.

Burchfield, S. R. (1979). The stress response: A new perspective. *Psychosomatic Medicine, 41,* 661–672.

Butler, S. R., Suskind, M. R., & Schanberg, S. M. (1978). Maternal behavior as a regulator of polyamine biosynthesis in brain and heart of the developing rat pup. *Science, 199,* 445–446.

Calvo, W. (1968). The innervation of the bone marrow in laboratory animals. *American Journal of Anatomy, 123,* 315–328.

Cappel, R., Gregoire, F., Thiry, L., Sprecher, S. (1978). Antibody and cell mediated immunity to Herpes simplex virus in psychotic depression. *Journal of Clinical Psychiatry, 39,* 266–268.

Claman, H. N. (1972). Cortiocosteroids and lymphoid cells. *New England Journal of Medicine, 287,* 388–397.

Clayton, P. J. (1979). The sequelae and nonsequelae of conjugal bereavement. *American Journal of Psychiatry, 136,* 1530–1534.

Clayton, P. J., Halikes, J. A., & Maurice, W..L. (1972). The depression of widowhood. *British Journal of Psychiatry, 120,* 71–78.

Coe, C. L., Mendoza, S. P., Smotherman, W. P., & Levine, S. (1978). Mother-infant attachment in the squirrel monkey: Adrenal response to separation. *Behavioral Biology, 22,* 256–263.

Cross, R. J., Brooks, W. H., Roszman, T. L., & Markesbery, R. (1982). Hypothalamic-immune interactions. Effect of hypophysectomy on neuroimmunomodulation. *Journal of the Neurological Sciences, 53,* 557–566.

Deberdt, R., Van Hooren, J., Biesbrouck, M., & Avery, W. (1976). Antinuclear factor-positive mental depression: A single disease entity. *Biological Psychiatry, 11,* 69–74.

Denckla, W. D. (1978). Interactions between age and neuroendocrine and immune systems. *Federation Proceedings, 37,* 1263–1266.

Endicott, J., Cohen, J., Nee, J., Fleiss, J., & Sarantakos, S. (1981). Hamilton depression rating scale. *Archives of General Psychiatry, 38,* 98–103.

Fauci, A. S. (1975). Cortiocosteroids and circulating lymphocytes. *Transplant Procedures, 7,* 37–48.

Fauci, A. S., & Dale, D. C. (1975). The effect of hydrocortisone on the kinetics of normal human lymphocytes. *Blood, 46,* 235–243.

Friedman, S. B., Glasgow, L. A., & Ader, R. (1969). Psychosocial factors modifying host resistance to experimental infections. *Annals of the New York Academy of Sciences, 164,* 381–382.

Gilman, S. C., Schwartz, J. M., Milner, R. J., Bloom, F. E., & Feldman, J. D. (1982). Endorphin enhances lymphocyte proliferative responses. *Proceedings of the National Academy of Science USA, 79,* 4226–4230.

Giron, L. T., Crutcher, K. A., & Davis, J. N. (1980). Lymph nodes—a possible site for sympathetic neuronal regulation of immune responses. *Annals of Neurology, 8,* 520–555.

Goodwin, J. S., Messner, R. P., & Williams, R. C. (1979). Inhibitors of T cell mitogenesis: Effect of mitogen dose. *Cellular Immunology, 45,* 303–308.

Harlow, C. M., & Selye, H. (1937). The blood picture in the alarm reaction. *Proceedings of the Society of Experimental Biology in Medicine, 36,* 141–144.

Helsing, K. J., Szklo, M., & Comstock, G. W. (1981). Factors associated with mortality after widowhood. *American Journal of Public Health, 71,* 802–809.

Hofer, M. A. (1981). Toward a developmental basis for disease predisposition: The effects of early maternal separation on brain, behavior, and cardiovascular system. In H. Weiner, M. A. Hofer, & A. J. Stunkard (Eds.), *Brain, behavior, and bodily disease* (pp. 209–228). New York: Raven Press.

Hofer, M. A., Wolff, C. T., Friedman, S. B., & Mason, J. W. (1972). A psychoendocrine study of bereavement, Part 2: Observations on the process of mourning in relation to adrenocortical function. *Psychosomatic Medicine, 34,* 492–504.

Jensen, M. M. (1969). Changes in leukocyte counts associated with various stressors. *Journal of the Reticuloendothelial Society, 6,* 457–465.

Jones, M. T., Hillhouse, E., & Burden, J. (1976). Secretion of cortiocotropin-releasing hormone in vivo. In L. Hartini & W. F. Ganong (Eds.), *Frontiers in neuroendocrinology* (Vol. 4). New York: Raven Press.

Keller, S. E., Ackerman, S., Schleifer, S. J., Shindledecker, R., Camerino, M. A., Hofer, M., Weiner, H., & Stein, M. (1983). Effect of premature weaning on lymphocyte stimulation in the rat. *Psychosomatic Medicine, 45*, 75.

Keller, S. E., Stein, M., Camerino, M. S., Schleifer, S. J., & Sherman, J. (1980). Suppression of lymphocyte stimulation by anterior hypothalamic lesions in the guinea pig. *Cellular Immunology, 52*, 334–340.

Keller, S. E., Weiss, J., Schleifer, S., Miller, N. E., & Stein, M. (1981). Suppression of immunity by stress: Effect of a graded series of stressors on lymphocyte stimulation in the rat. *Science, 213*, 1397–1400.

Keller, S. E., Weiss, J. M., Schleifer, S. J., Miller, N. E., & Stein, M. (1983). Stress-induced suppression of immunity in adrenalectomized rats. *Science, 221*, 1301–1304.

Kronfol, Z., Silva, J., Jr., Greden, J.,Dembinski, S., Gardner, R., & Carroll, B. (1983). Impaired lymphocyte function in depressive illness. *Life Sciences, 33*, 241–247.

Kuhn, C. M., Butler, S. R., & Schanberg, S. M. (1978). Selective depression of serum growth hormone during maternal deprivation in rat pups. *Science, 201*, 1034–1036.

Marsh, J. T., & Rasmussen, A. F. (1960). Response of adrenal, thymus, spleen, and leukocytes to shuttle box and confinement stress. *Proceedings of the Society of Experimental Biology in Medicine, 104*, 180–183.

Meyer, E. M., Meyer, G., Niehaus, W., Schlake, E., & Grundmann, E. (1980). Divergence of cortisol-induced involution of T and B cells areas in mouse lymph nodes and spleen. A histomorphometrical, enzyme-histochemical, and immunohistochemical study. *Investigations in Cell Pathology, 3*, 175–180.

Michaut, R. J., Dechambre, R. P., Doumerc, S., Lesourd, B., Devillechabrolle, A., & Moulias, R. (1981). Influence of early maternal deprivation on adult humoral immune response in mice. *Physiology and Behavior, 26*, 189–191.

Palmblad, J., Petrini, B., Wasserman, J., & Akerstedt, T. (1979). Lymphocyte and granulocyte reactions during sleep deprivation. *Psychosomatic Medicine, 41*, 273–278.

Parkes, C. M. (1972). *Bereavement: Studies of grief in adult life*. New York: International University Press.

Pochet, R., Delesperse, G., Gauseet, P. W., & Collet, H. (1979). Distribution of beta-adrenergic receptors on human lymphocyte subpopulations. *Clinical Experimental Immunology, 38*, 578–584.

Riley, M. W. (in press). Aging, health, and social change. In M. W. Riley, A. S. Baum, & J. D. Matarazzo (Eds.), *Perspectives on behavioral medicine: Vol. IV. Biomedical and psychosocial dimensions of aging*. Hillsdale, NJ: Lawrence Erlbaum Associates.

Riley, V. (1981). Psychoneuroendocrine influences on immunocompetence and neoplasia. *Science, 212*, 1100–1109.

Roess, D. A., Bellone, M. F., Ruh, M. F., Nadel, E. M., & Ruh, E. M. (1982). The effect of glucocorticoids on mitogen-stimulated B-lymphocytes: Thymidine incorporation and Ab secretion. *Endocrinology, 110*, 169–175.

Schleifer, S. J., Keller, S. E., Camerino, M., Thornton, J. C., & Stein, M. (1983). Suppression of lymphocyte stimulation following bereavement. *Journal of the American Medical Association, 250*, 374–377.

Schleifer, S. J., Keller, S. E., Meyerson, A. T., Raskin, M. J., Davis, K. L., & Stein, M. (1984). Lymphocyte function in major depressive disorder. *Archives of General Psychiatry, 41*, 483–486.

Schleifer, S. J., Keller, S. E., Siris, S. G., Davis, K. L., & Stein, M. (1985). Depression and immunity. Lymphocyte function in ambulatory depressed, hospitalized schizophrenic, and herniorrhaphy patients. *Archives of General Psychiatry, 42*, 129–133.

Schleifer, S. J., Keller, S. E., & Stein, M. (1984). Brain, behaviour and the immune system [letter to the editor]. *Nature, 310*, 456.

Selye, H. (1976). *Stress in health and disease.* Boston: Butterworths.

Shavit, Y., Lewis, J. W., Terman, G. W., Gale, R. P., & Liebeskind, J. C. (1984). Opioid peptides mediate the suppressive effect of stress on natural killer cell cytotoxicity. *Science, 223*, 188–190.

Sherman, N. A., Smith, R. S., & Middleton, E., Jr. (1973). Effect of adrenergic compounds, aminophylline and hydrocortisone, on in vitro immunoglobulin synthesis by normal human peripheral lymphocytes. *Journal of Allergy and Clinical Immunology, 52*, 13–22.

Shopsin, B., Sathananthan, G. L., Chan, T. L., Kravitz, H., Gershon, S. (1973). Antinuclear factor in psychiatric patients. *Biological Psychiatry, 7*, 81–86.

Smith, E. M., Meyer, W. J., & Blalock, J. E. (1982). Virus-induced corticosterone in hypophysectomized mice: A possible lymphoid adrenal axis. *Science, 218*, 1311–1312.

Spitzer, R. L., Endicott, J., & Robins, E. (1978). Research diagnostic criteria: Rationale and reliability. *Archives of General Psychiatry, 35*, 773–782.

Stein, M., Keller, S., & Schleifer, S. (1981). The hypothalamus and the immune response. In H. Weiner, M. A. Hofer, & A. J. Stunkard (Eds.), *Brain, behavior and bodily disease* (pp. 45–65). New York: Raven Press.

Stein, M., Schleifer, S., & Keller, S. (1982). The role of the brain and neuroendocrine system in immune regulation: Potential links to neoplastic disease. In S. Levy (Ed.), *Biological mediators of behavior and disease* (pp. 147–168). New York: Elsevier North Holland.

Tache, Y., DuRuisseau, P., Tache, J., Selye, H., & Collu, R. (1976). Shift in adrenohypophyseal activity during chronic intermittent immobilization of rats. *Neuroendocrinology, 22*, 325–336.

Tavadia, H. B., Fleming, K. A., Hume, R. D., & Simpson, H. (1975). Circadian rhythmicity of human plasma cortisol and PHA-induced lymphocyte transformation. *Clinical Experimental Immunology, 22*, 190–193.

Tennenbaum, J. I., Ruppert, R. D., St. Pierre, R. L., & Greenberger, N. (1969). The effect of chronic alcohol administration on the immune responsiveness of rats. *Journal of Allergy, 44*, 272–281.

Thomson, S. P., McMahon, L. J., & Nugent, C. A. (1980). Endogenous cortisol: A regulator of the number of lymphocytes in peripheral blood. *Clinical Immunology and Immunopathology, 17*, 506–514.

Williams, J. W., Peterson, R. G., Shea, P. A., Schmedtje, J. F., Bauer, D. C., & Felton, D. L. (1980). Sympathetic innervation of murine thymus and spleen: Evidence for a functional link between the nervous and immune systems. *Brain Research Bulletin, 6*, 83–94.

9

INTERVENTIONS AND AGING

A Note on Biomedical Perspective

Edward L. Schneider
National Institute on Aging

Two ancient dreams of mankind have been to be wealthy and to live forever. Thus, two of the earliest areas of scientific endeavor were alchemy and gerontology. Fortunes have been squandered on schemes for achieving instant wealth and for obtaining continuous youth. Today, billions of dollars are spent annually on cosmetics, vitamins, food supplements, and other items advertised to preserve youth and prevent aging.

Unfortunately, biomedical scientists have not been particularly interested in searching for interventions related to aging or even in evaluating proposed interventions. (For a fuller treatment, see Schneider & Reid, 1985.) There are several reasons behind this lack of enthusiasm by the scientific community. Probably the most important contributing factor has been the general lack of interest in gerontological research by the biomedical community. Another important factor is the pessimism of scientists concerning the possibilities of successful interventions. Finally, there are those who feel that extension of life span would have negative consequences for society. Thus, we have abdicated the area of interventions in aging to fringe scientists. In this paper we will address these issues and examine potential interventions.

The lack of interest in biomedical gerontological research has dissipated in the last few years. This may have been catalyzed by the creation of the National Institute on Aging (NIA) and the Geriatric Research Education Clinical Centers (GRECC) by the Veterans Administration (VA). As a result, we have witnessed an exponential increase in the number of investigators in the field of aging research. Pessimism concerning aging has greatly influenced the attitudes of physicians and scientists toward aging research. If you look at aging as a series of immutable, unalterable losses of functions, it is not surprising that you might consider intervention related to aging as a futile exercise. However, a historical perspective indicates that a similar pessimism about interventions in cancer existed 20 years ago. Few if any cancers were curable at that time. Now, several cancers are 100% curable, and there is considerable interest in searching for new interventive approaches in oncology.

Are we facing a biologic limit to life span? If there is a fixed genetically determined life span, interventions in aging might have limited impact. Fries (1980) has postulated that we are rapidly approaching maximum human life expectancy at approximately 85 years. However, examination of actuarial data indicates that maximum life expectancy has been increasing and that these increases will not stop at an 85-year limit (Schneider & Brody, 1983).

Proponents of the competitive risk theory suggest that as one age-related disease is controlled, others will increase in frequency to negate any significant increases in life span. However, examination of mortality trends in the last two decades does not support this contention. While cardiovascular mortality, the leading cause of death, has declined 12% in individuals over age 65 since 1965 (Kovar, 1977), deaths from cancer, the second leading cause of death, have shown only a modest 1% increase in this period (Schneiderman, 1979). There has not been a compensatory increase in other diseases to replace cardiovascular disease. Instead, individuals over age 65 have experienced an increase in life expectancy, and the absolute number of deaths after ages 65, 75, and even 85, is declining (Brody & Brock, 1985).

It has been suggested that there may be a genetically determined biological limit to life span in man (Fries, 1980). This argument was based on the observation that human fetal lung fibroblasts, when placed into tissue culture, have a finite number of cell replications (Hayflick & Moorhead, 1961). However, it has been demonstrated that replicating cell populations in vivo survive well past the life span of the organism (Daniel & Young, 1971; Harrison, 1973). Thus, it is highly unlikely that the in vivo survival of the organism is related to the limited replicating ability of cells in tissue culture.

The remarkable achievements of modern medicine, such as the introduction of antibiotics and vaccines for the conquest of infectious diseases, have encouraged the hope for "magic bullets" for other diseases. Many of the theories proposed to explain biologic aging have focused on a single mechanism, thus encouraging research to find a single "magic bullet" to arrest aging. Progress in cancer research, where a "magic bullet" has been sought intensively for decades, points toward multiple etiologies for various malignancies. Thus, it is becoming increasingly probable that multiple interventions will be necessary to prevent and/or cure various malignancies. Our current knowledge of the mechanisms of aging is clearly at an earlier stage than cancer research. In aging research, as in cancer research, increasing knowledge should reveal multiple mechanisms underlying aging processes at the molecular, cellular, and organ levels. Therefore, I predict that it is equally unlikely that a single "magic bullet" will reverse or arrest all aging processes.

While it is unlikely that a single intervention will affect all aging processes, segmental interventions (interventions which affect one organ system) may be developed which have significant impacts on specific aging processes. An example would be the potential attempt to prevent or restore the decline in immune function that occurs with aging or to slow or arrest the bone loss in postmenopausal women. These segmental interventions can best be assessed through the measurements of specific biomarkers of aging. The proceedings of a NIA conference which examined various segmental interventions in rodents and humans has been published (Reff & Schneider, 1982).

What are the biological risks of interventions into aging processes? The immune system provides an example of the potential risks of interventions to alter aging processes. The age-related decline in the function of the immune system may have evolved as a beneficial mechanism. Since an increase in autoimmune phenomena occurs with aging, the decline in immune function may protect us from the development of high levels of autoimmune diseases in old age. Restoring immune function to youthful levels might potentially increase the incidence of autoimmune diseases in older individuals. Thus, any attempts to intervene in aging processes should carefully consider the risks of potential adverse responses.

In addition to the biological considerations for life extension, there are important ethical considerations. In the literature, fictional characters have exchanged their souls for perpetual youth with unfortunate consequences. Are the increases in life expectancy a mixed blessing? Will they produce more harm than good for the individual and society?

The addition of years of dependency, illness, and disability would certainly not be a blessing to the individual or to society. However, the vast majority of our older citizens enter their last decades without significant disability. The addition of healthy years clearly should not be considered detrimental to this group. Society should also benefit from the addition of productive, healthy years to its mature and elderly population. Therefore, interventions to increase longevity should be oriented to the maintenance of health and vigor, rather than to prolonging terminal illnesses.

Interventions which modify aging processes may also contribute to changing the biases which exist in relation to aging. Many of the negative feelings about aging are derived from the concept that aging is the sum of a series of losses of individual functions. Thus, many physicians conceive that their role is mostly supportive of the elderly patient. Successful segmental interventions (Reff & Schneider, 1982), which arrest or even reverse the aging of certain organs, would demonstrate that some declines in function may not be inevitable and thus provide a positive stimulus for increasing the interest of physicians in caring for the elderly.

A wide range of environmental, chemical, hormonal, and pharmacological interventions have been examined for their ability to extend life span and to arrest aging processes in a variety of organisms (Table 9.1). These interventions are extensively examined elsewhere (Schneider & Reed, 1985). In this paper we will discuss a few of these interventions. The intervention that has most consistently been demonstrated in animals to increase longevity and to affect the largest range of aging processes is caloric restriction. Of particular interest is the observation that this intervention can be successful even if commenced at mid-life in experimental animals.

Skeptics have suggested that caloric restriction is the natural state of organisms that feed on an irregular schedule. Therefore, the caged ad-libitum-fed laboratory rodent, which has been used for most studies of caloric restriction, may be an overweight animal with an abnormal feeding schedule. This argument is unresolvable since comparative life span studies on wild mice and rats could not be conducted in their natural environment which is filled with predators. It is of interest that many of the other interventions that have been reported to increase life span produce weight loss. In Table 9.2, the presence or absence of weight loss is listed for some of the interventions that have been claimed to increase mean or maximum life span. Thus, the proposed life-extending properties of many of these interventions may be related to caloric restriction.

While the effects of caloric restriction are impressive in rodents, it is too early to suggest this approach as a possible intervention in man. The caged ad-libitum-fed mouse may not be an appropriate model for the free-living human population. In addition, review of the data accumulated by life insurance companies suggests that being moderately overweight rather than underweight may be correlated with increased life span (Andres, 1981). However, the definitions of ideal body weight used for these studies were low and have subsequently been increased. Therefore, at this time there is little advice that can be given to individuals concerning the optimum caloric intake for longevity.

TABLE 9.1
Interventions Proposed to Alter Life Span

Caloric restriction
Hypothermia
Exercise
Antioxidants
Vitamins
Superoxide Dismutase
Centrophenoxine
L-dopa
Hypophysectomy
Coenzyme Q
Thymosin
DHEA
Gerovital

TABLE 9.2
Relation Between Weight Loss and Effects of Various Interventions on
Life Span and Age-Related Changes in Rodents

Intervention	Prolongs Life Span	Prevents or Delays Age-Related Changes	Weight Loss
L-dopa	Yes	Yes	Yes
Antioxidants	Yes	–	Yes/No
Vitamin E	Yes	Yes	Yes/No
Centrophenoxine	Yes	Yes	Yes
Hypophysectomy	Yes	Yes	Yes
DHEA	Yes	Yes	Yes

Future segmental interventions may focus on cholinergic neurons. The proposed cholinergic deficit that accompanies aging has been summarized in an extensive review (Bartus, Dean, Beer, & Lippa, 1982). This decline in cholinergic activity may be associated with age-related memory changes. The administration of choline was demonstrated to reverse the age-related decline in memory observed in laboratory rodents (Bartus et al., 1982).

An accelerated decline in cholinergic function is also postulated to be involved in senile dementia of the Alzheimer's type (Bartus et al., 1982). Pharmacologic interventions to restore cholinergic function could involve administration of acetylcholine precursors, cholinergic agonists, and acetylcholinesterase inhibitors. This approach has been successful in Parkinson's disease, which features a loss of dopaminergic neurons in the substantia nigra. Oral administration of L-dopa, a precursor of dopamine, has been effective in diminishing the symptoms of this disorder (Rinne, Sonninen, & Siirtola, 1972).

Another promising approach for the future is through the transplantation of cholinergic neurons to brain areas that have lost significant numbers of cholinergic neurons. The brain is a good site for transplantation since blood-brain barriers may slow or reduce immune rejection of the transplanted tissues. Several investigators have demonstrated that transplanted fetal brain tissue can function effectively in the adult recipient brain (Krieger et al., 1982).

A promising segmental intervention is exercise, which may have significant effects on slowing age-related changes in glucose metabolism, bone loss, and cardiovascular function. The effect of exercise on cardiac function is of particular interest. It has been demonstrated in rats that several of the cardiac parameters which declined with aging could be significantly slowed by exercise.

Application of many interventions may have to wait for gerontologic research to progress to the point where logical applications are possible. Aging research, while one of the oldest areas of research interest, has had substantial financial support only in the last ten years. Therefore, it is not surprising that we know relatively little about the basic mechanisms of aging at the molecular, cellular, and organ levels. Until our knowledge of these areas is more complete, formulation of effective interventions may be very difficult. Major efforts should therefore continue to be focused on basic research to elucidate the mechanisms of aging processes.

The future for segmental interventions is extremely promising. The exciting developments in molecular biology, immunology, endocrinology, and the neurosciences should lead to effective segmental interventions. These interventions will need to be rigorously tested with standardized biomarkers of aging in appropriate animal models and then examined in carefully designed, well-controlled human clinical studies. Until then, caution will need to be exercised in dealing with claims for rejuvenating properties of various agents or regimens.

REFERENCES

Andres, R. (1981). Aging, diabetes, and obesity: Standards of normality. *Mount Sinai Journal of Medicine, 48,* 489–495.

Bartus, T. R., Dean, R. L., III, Beer, B., & Lippa, A. S. (1982). The cholinergic hypothesis of geriatric memory dysfunction. *Science, 217,* 408–417.

Brody, J. A., & Brock, D. B. (1985). Epidemiologic and statistical characterizations of the United States' elderly population. In C. Finch & E. L. Schneider (Eds.), *Handbook of the biology of aging* (2nd ed., pp. 3–26). New York: Van Nostrand Reinhold.

Daniel, C. W., & Young, L. J. T. (1971). Influence of cell division on an aging process. Life span of mouse mammary epithelium during serial propagation *in vivo. Experimental Cell Research, 65,* 27–32.

Fries, J. F. (1980). Aging, natural death, and the compression of morbidity. *New England Journal of Medicine, 303,* 130–135.

Harrison, D. E. (1973). Normal production of erythrocytes by mouse marrow continuous for 73 months. *Proceedings of the National Academy of Sciences, (USA), 11,* 3184–3188.

Hayflick, L., & Moorhead, P. S. (1961). The serial cultivation of human diploid cell strains. *Experimental Cell Research, 65,* 27–32.

Kovar, M. G. (1977). Elderly people: The population 65 years and over. In *Health, United States, 1976–1977* (pp. 3–26). Washington, D.C.: DHEW Publication No. (HRA) 77–1232.

Krieger, D. T., Perlow, M. J., Gibson, M. J., Davies, T. F., Zimmerman, E. A., Ferin, M., & Charlton, H. M. (1982). Brain grafts reverse hypogonadism of gonadotropin releasing hormone deficiency. *Nature, 298,* 468–471.

Reff, M. E., & Schneider, E. L. (1982). *Biological markers of aging* Washington, D.C.: U.S. Health and Human Services Publication No. 82–2221.

Rinne, U. K., Sonninen, V., & Siirtola, T. (1972). Treatment of Parkinson's disease with L-dopa and a decarboxylase inhibitor. *Journal of Neurology, 202,* 1–20.

Schneider, E. L., Brody, J. A. (1983). Aging, natural death, and the compression of morbidity: Another view. *New England Journal of Medicine, 309,* 854–856.

Schneider, E. L., & Reed, J. D., Jr. (1985). Modulations of aging processes. In C. Finch & E. L. Schneider (Eds.), *Handbook of the biology of aging* (2nd ed., pp. 45–76). New York: Van Nostrand Reinhold.

Schneiderman, M. A. (1979, March 5). *A statement by Marvin A. Schneiderman, Ph.D., National Cancer Institute, on trends in cancer incidence and mortality in the United States.* Subcommittee on Health and Scientific Research, Senate Committee on Human Resources.

10

INTERVENTION AND AGING
Enrichment and Prevention

Judith Rodin
Cheryl Cashman
Laurie Desiderato
Yale University

There are two important assumptions being made in a paper dealing with psychosocial interventions in aging. The first is that it is possible to intervene in ways that can reverse or alter factors thought to be associated with the aging process per se or with common experiences to which most older people are exposed. The second is that these interventions can be psychosocial in nature, that is, manipulating psychological, behavioral, or environmental variables rather than biomedical ones. We contend that there is some evidence for both of these important assertions, although surprisingly the data are far less persuasive than one might suspect, given the great enthusiasm for the possibility of intervention that has been expressed in the field (cf. Fozard & Popkin, 1978; Poon, Fozard, & Treat, 1978). Our examination of the literature revealed that several of the intervention studies lack outcome measures, making it impossible to evaluate whether many of the very interesting approaches that have been tried actually have any measurable, not to mention clinically significant, effects. Furthermore, most intervention studies in this area lack a conceptual view of the process of aging, and almost all of them fail to take what we would characterize as a biopsychosocial approach.

TAXONOMY OF INTERVENTIONS

To evaluate the limited number of intervention studies with true outcome measures, we first looked for a way to organize them. Table 10.1 presents a schema suggested by Baltes (1973), based on an earlier categorization by Jacobs (1972).

TABLE 10.1
Parameters of Psychological Intervention Strategies: Examples

Goal	Target behavior	Setting	Mechanism
Enrichment	Cognition	Laboratory	Training—practice
Prevention	Language	Family	Social learning
Alleviation	Intellectual abilities	Classroom	Psychotherapy
	Social interactions	Senior citizen center	Environmenal change
	Motivational states	Hospital	Health delivery
	Personality traits	Community	Economic support
	Attitudes	Macroecology	

It suggests organizing studies on the basis of their goal, the target behavior to be changed, the mechanism to effect the change, and the setting in which the intervention takes place. Its orientation on these parameters is pragmatic in that it attempts to focus on the diversity of possible intervention activities.

The cognitive domain has been one of the major areas in which intervention efforts have been made, with studies trying to influence memory and intellectual abilities in particular. A second area that has been targeted is social interaction. Based on a substantial number of correlational studies, which suggest that social activity and social support decline with advancing age, work has been done to try to bolster social support and increase the interaction of older people, (Kahn & Antonnucci, 1981). The third broad area of intervention focuses on changing the individual's thoughts and feelings, looking at motivational states, personality traits, and attitudes.

Most interesting to us in this taxonomy is the way that general intervention goals have been described not only in terms of correcting or preventing dysfunction, but also from the perspective of maximizing human potential. Thus the term "enrichment" introduces a new dimension and concept, which involves the optimization of human development throughout the life span.

In an excellent review, Gatz, Popkin, Pino, and VandenBos (1985) focused particularly on alleviation interventions, and, indeed, most gerontological intervention has concentrated thus far on alleviation of seemingly deficient behaviors rather than on prevention or enrichment. Gatz et al. (1985) heavily emphasized psychotherapy as the prototypical psychological intervention, but also reviewed nontraditional (e.g., pet therapy) and institutional alleviation programs. So as not to duplicate efforts, our review will focus especially on the prevention and enrichment interventions. These also have greater theoretical interest for us because they imply even more strongly than alleviation approaches that there is a great deal of plasticity in the system, that life-span development is a process, and that optimization of function is possible. In essence, we see the effort to optimize function as an opportunity to ask questions regarding the malleability of bodily systems as they age. By choosing terms like "prevention," "enrichment," and "optimization," there is the intent to convey that aging is a process. It is not a static event, but rather involves an interaction of the person's current physical and mental state with past states and present experiences. Intervention efforts, therefore, must be process-oriented, in order to be maximally effective.

This taxonomic effort also implies a relationship between the intervention and the theoretical context formulated for the target of the intervention efforts. Enrichment, prevention, and alleviation all presuppose some implicit or explicit theory of the natural or the desirable state or course of the target phenomenon.

THEMES APPEARING REPEATEDLY
IN INTERVENTION STUDIES

From our perspective, four major themes emerge after reviewing the literature on psychosocial interventions in aging. Let us highlight these so as to put the review of the studies themselves in perspective. First, there is a tremendous amount of evidence suggesting plasticity in the aging process. While there is little doubt that there is some real decline in health and function with aging, the more relevant question is whether we understand the multiple factors that are producing what declines we see. And if we can understand those converging sets of factors, can we intervene in some effective way? The answer seems to be "yes." Plasticity certainly stands out as one of the main themes in reviewing this literature.

A second theme is between-subject variability in responses, variability that seems to increase with age rather than decrease. While it was once thought that there was greater variability at the early stages of life, much of the data actually suggest quite the opposite—that there is much less variability among newborns than persons at the other end of the age continuum. This finding is not surprising as long as we take an interactionist view of human development, thus predicting that the variability would only tend to increase throughout the life span.

A third theme is the concept of control or efficacy, which emerges very strongly in this area. The Gatz et al. (1985) review of alleviation studies concluded that expectancy and efficacy appear to be changed by virtually every type of successful therapeutic intervention with older adults. Psychotherapy that combats helplessness and demoralization certainly appears most effective (Frank, 1976). Our review reaches the same conclusion regarding prevention and enrichment interventions.

The importance of perceived efficacy in effecting change is relevant to the fourth theme that emerges in this literature. It is very clear that how the aid is delivered can be a major determinant of whether people first seek help, continue to accept help, and how they feel after receiving it. The helping process can be undermined if the helper takes on too much responsibility for generating and implementing all of the solutions, or if the helper and the recipient have incongruent attributions about who is responsible for what (Brickman et al., 1982). A consequence of discrepant perception may be a service provision system where the act of helping is rendered in a fashion that reduces the older person's sense of control and sense of self-esteem (Gatz et al., 1985). Therefore the nature of the helping process as these interventions unfold seems to be a very important determinant of their long-range efficacy.

COGNITIVE INTERVENTIONS

One kind of intervention that has been widely used involves reminiscence. The assumption in these studies is that reminiscence involves a set of cognitive operations; for example, it requires raw data to be taken from past memory and then organized and reconstructed to present and provide some information to people about past history. It is not the accuracy of the material that is important, but the exercise in mental function that is required to deal with this material.

Hughston and Merriam (1982) randomly assigned 105 community residents to three treatment conditions. One group received an intervention involving reminiscence in structured groups. Subjects in a second condition were required to learn a variety of new materials, for example to memorize lists of names. They met in the group context for an equal amount of time as the reminiscence group. Finally there was a no-treatment group. Table 10.2 presents changes in cognitive function measured by the Raven Standard Progressive Matrices (five sets of increasingly difficult problems testing a person's capacity for intellectual functioning). While the reminiscence group did only marginally better than the "new material" group, both groups performed significantly better than the no-treatment controls. When the sexes were looked at separately, females were

TABLE 10.2
Mean Pretest and Posttest Scores on the Raven, by Method and Sex

Method			Pretest $\bar{X}$	S.D.	Posttest $\bar{X}$	S.D.	Mean Change
A (New material)	7	Male	33.57	13.94	35.00	11.87	+1.43
	20	Female	37.15	15.76	38.10	14.09	+0.95
	27	Combined	36.22	15.13	37.30	13.39	+1.08
B (Reminiscence)	6	Male	29.83	16.18	28.67	15.53	−1.16
	22	Female	35.81	12.81	39.50	13.58	+3.69
	28	Combined	34.54	13.50	36.82	14.89	+2.28
C (Control)	7	Male	32.43	13.62	31.43	11.91	−1.00
	21	Female	31.80	16.31	29.71	15.78	−2.09
	28	Combined	31.96	15.44	30.14	14.71	−1.82

significantly benefited by reminiscence as compared to memorizing new material. It may be that for women, at least in this study, there was some added benefit from talking about the past, which may have had a stronger effect on motivating intellectual performance than it did for men.

In another study in this domain, Perrotta and Meacham (1981–1982) also tested a reminiscence manipulation, which they compared to a no-treatment control group. Subjects were elderly people who lived in the community, who were randomly assigned to condition. The authors did not use cognitive measures, asking instead whether reminiscence generalizes to other behaviors that might be important and beneficial for older persons. They measured self-esteem and reduction in depression, and they found weak effects of the reminiscence manipulation, with no effects in the other two groups. Unfortunately, the small number of subjects ($n = 21$) prevented a strong test of their intervention procedure.

Another group of studies has considered how cognitive intervention might influence memory in older persons. There is ample evidence of age differences in acquisition of new information (Craik, 1977). Some procedures that improve acquisition and subsequent recall include teaching organizational strategies like putting a word list into categories (Hultsch, 1969, 1975) and the use of verbal or visual mediators to make connections between pairs of words (Canestrari, 1968; Hulicka & Grossman, 1967; Treat & Reese, 1976).

Zarit, Cole, and Guider (1981) asked whether instruction in memory enhancement would affect a variety of tasks that are increasingly more unrelated to the teaching task. Subjects in the memory training group were taught organizational strategies, mnemonic devices of one sort or another, and imagery techniques. Figure 10.1 shows data at the pre-intervention time point, the post-measure immediately following the intervention, and a one-month follow-up. On the test items closest to the training, subjects who were given memory training showed substantial improvement compared to the waiting-list control group. They also were significantly different on the next most-related items and on the group of unrelated items placed in the context of a similar task. However, the most-different kind of task showed virtually no effect at all of the intervention. Thus, there are two conclusions from this study. One is that it is possible to show improvement in memory as a result of specific interventions that focus on teaching cognitive skills, but second it appears that the more distant one gets from the actual training task, the less effect one has on performance.

Zarit and coworkers were also interested in whether these kinds of interventions improved subjective memory. The data are fairly clear that when older persons are questioned about their memory performance, they rate themselves as substantially poorer than they actually perform. Thus it is a common finding that older persons perform better on memory tasks than their self-evaluation would indicate (Gurland et al., 1976; Kahn, Zarit, Hilbert, & Niederehe, 1975; Lowenthal, Thurner, & Chiriboga, 1975; Perlmutter, 1978). Interestingly, this effect is even stronger when the older persons are depressed (Kahn et al., 1975).

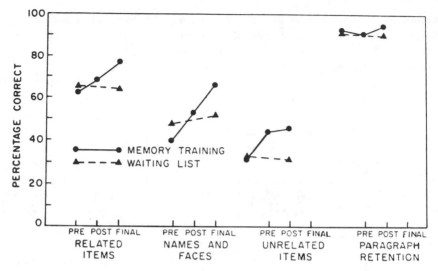

FIGURE 10.1   Percentage of items correct on test items from left to right that were increasingly different from training items (from Zarit, Cole, & Gurder, 1981).

These findings, however, do not suggest the direction of the effect. For example, an older person might simply make more of having forgotten something than would a younger person who forgot the same thing. Thus, any evidence of memory loss is far more salient for an older person (cf. Taylor & Fiske, 1978). It is therefore significant that the memory training not only affected actual performance in the Zarit et al. (1981) study but that prior to the performance measures, the intervention showed a very strong effect on subjective memory. Subjects in the training group reported feeling that they could do better and, in fact, they did. Obviously these are simply correlational data, but they suggest some interesting ideas for potential interventions. It appears to us that subjects' perceived efficacy with regard to memory performance was increased by the intervention, thus leading to the observed improvements.

In a different study, Plemons, Willis, & Baltes (1978) examined training of intelligence based on Cattell and Horn's theories (Horn, 1972, 1978; Horn & Cattell, 1967). This study is a model intervention study because it used a theory as a conceptual framework to provide both a systematic definition of the appropriate cognitive intervention targets and of transfer of training measures. Fluid intelligence is the ability to deal with essentially new problems, whereas crystallized intelligence is the repertoire of information, cognitive skills, and strategies that is developed by the individual by applying his or her fluid intelligence. Plemons et al. (1978) suggested that fluid intelligence may decline with age, but that crystallized intelligence may not.

Plemons et al. (1978) attempted to teach skills that would improve an individual's fluid intelligence. Subjects were randomly assigned to condition and given eight practice sessions using Figure Relations items, which require the subjects to identify relations between figures in a pattern and produce one element missing from it (Horn, 1972). As were Zarit et al. (1981), these investigators were asking two major questions: Did the training maintain itself and for how long? How different could the task be and still show important intervention effects? Training effectiveness was thus assessed by its duration and by its effect on a hierarchical set of transfer measures. Figure 10.2 shows their results. In

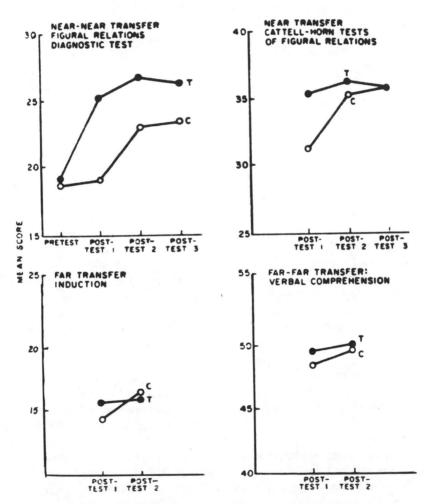

FIGURE 10.2.   Mean number of items correct on test items measured prior to, and at three time points following training. Starting in upper left panel and going to the lower right panel, the test items are increasingly different from the training items (from Plemons, Willis, & Baltes, 1978).

the panel labeled "near-near transfer," which is the same kind of test as the training although with different figures, data are presented from a series of tests. Post-test 1 is immediately after the training, post-test 2 is two months later, and post-test 3 is six months later.

As Figure 10.2 reveals, for the "near-near" transfer test, subjects in the training group were no different from controls at pre-test, but they did substantially better at the immediate post-test. While the effect decreased somewhat over time, the differences between groups seemed to maintain themselves over the six-month interval. The remaining three panels represented tests that were increasingly different from the training task. On all three tasks, experimental subjects did better than controls, but these effects were gone by the six-month post-test.

From these data we might conclude that there is some effect of the intervention when it is comparable to the training task and the effects tend to maintain themselves over time, but that the further the task is from the intervention, the more difficult it is both to show an effect and also to get those effects to maintain themselves. Thus the message is both good and bad. Some enrichment is possible, but it is clear from this study that the impact is not on a general cognitive system. Rather it seems to be fairly specific, which may be an analogue to biological systems. Further, the effects do not seem to maintain themselves.

An alternative conclusion would be based on the assumption that the efforts described thus far have been aimed at teaching cognitive skills directly with cognitive skills-kinds of interventions. That is, if we want someone to do better on a Figure Relations task, we teach them how to do Figure Relations problems. While conceptually that is certainly a sound approach, all that subjects may be learning from these enrichment efforts is a single skill and not one that is especially generalizable. Suppose we take a different view of what is influencing memory or cognitive skills in an aging person. Consider the speculation that memory and cognitive skills are not only attributable to intrinsic biological factors, but may also be strongly affected by environmental variables that may enhance or mask the real cognitive ability of older people.

How might social factors impact on cognitive processes? Many older people live in settings that are not environmentally challenging. For them, every day is like every other day, there is very little to remember, and there is very little to think about. Living in such highly redundant environments leaves one with little information to process and few incentives to try. As a result, the ability to think and remember may diminish. We questioned whether, by changing aspects of the environment, we might stimulate the desire to think, to interact with the environment, and to use whatever cognitive skills were available.

In one set of studies, we (Langer, Rodin, Beck, Weinman & Spitzer, 1977) attempted to motivate subjects to adhere to a recommended course of action over time that asked them to think about various issues. Commitment to increased cognitive activity was encouraged in the first study by providing the opportunity for reciprocal self-disclosure between the subject and an interviewer who recommended the particular course of cognitive activity.

According to Janis and Rodin (1979), eliciting self-disclosure and reciprocating with self-disclosure is one factor that is critical in helping a person to establish referent power (French & Raven, 1959) that promotes commitment to recommended courses of action. Persons have referent power for those who perceive them as likable, benevolent, admirable, and accepting. Their motivating power derives from this source. Janis and Rodin (1979) have described how the use of referent power in health care settings promotes internalization of medical recommendations made by health care professionals.

Langer et al. (1979) used a series of reciprocal self-disclosure conversations as an incentive for adhering to a particular course of recommended cognitive activity. The cognitive activity involved remembering a series of questions and searching the environment and one's long-term memory for information relevant to their answers. A low-self-disclosure group was included to control for the amount of time spent with an interviewer discussing past and present events. This more standard interview procedure, however, was not expected to provide sufficient interpersonal incentive to occasion the kind of commitment necessary to stimulate renewed cognitive activity. To control for changes that may have occurred simply because of multiple administrations of the memory tests, a no-treatment group was added to the design. We used pre- and post-measures of two different kinds of memory tests (pattern recall tests measuring memory for increasingly complex patterns and a paired-associates learning task).

The results of this study, shown in Tables 10.3 and 10.4, suggest that memory can be improved when the elderly are motivated to commit themselves to a recommended course of action that involves increased use of their cognitive abilities. Because people in the high reciprocal-self-disclosure group spoke more

TABLE 10.3
Mean Change Scores (Posttreatment Minus Pretreatment) on Memory
Tests for Each Experimental Condition as a Function of Level of
Involvement

| | Memory test | | | | | |
| | Pattern recall | | | Probe recall | | |
Group	Pre	Post	Change	Pre	Post	Change
High reciprocal self-disclosure	4.7	6.7	2.0$_a$	10.0	15.3	5.3$_a$
Low reciprocal self-disclosure	4.0	3.3	−.7$_b$	12.2	9.2	−3.0$_b$
No treatment	4.8	4.6	−.2$_b$	11.5	9.0	−2.5$_b$

Note: Different subscripts within each test indicate significiant differences at $p < .05$.

TABLE 10.4

Nurses' Mean Ratings (Posttreatment Minus Pretreatment Scores) of
Residents' Behavior by Experimental Condition

Group	Mood	Awareness	Sociability	Activity	Self-initiating	Alertness	Health
High reciprocal self-disclosure							
Pre	4.5	3.5	5.3	3.0	2.8	6.5	4.3
Post	5.0	5.8	7.0	4.5	5.3	6.8	5.1
Change	$.5_a$	2.3_a	1.7_a	1.5_a	2.5_a	$.3_a$	$.8_a$
Low reciprocal self-disclosure							
Pre	4.8	4.7	5.0	3.3	3.7	5.8	4.7
Post	5.5	5.2	4.5	1.7	5.7	5.8	4.7
Change	$.7_a$	$.5_b$	$-.5_a$	-1.6_b	2.0_a	$.0_a$	$.0_a$
No treatment							
Pre	4.0	4.5	5.3	3.8	3.5	5.8	4.0
Post	4.3	4.5	4.0	3.5	4.0	5.8	4.0
Change	$.3_a$	$.0_b$	-1.3_a	$-.3_b$	$.5_b$	$.0_a$	$.0_a$

Note: Cells bearing different subscripts within each rating are significantly different at $p < .05$.

and initiated more topics for conversation than their low self-disclosure coun-
terparts during the six-week period of the study, they appear to have been more
involved in the substance and conduct of the interviews. This greater involvement
apparently led to a greater commitment to follow the interviewer's recommendations to think about a variety of proposed topics for future discussion. Although
the low-involvement group also was asked to think about things to be discussed
in between the scheduled visits, the character of the interaction was not sufficiently involving to encourage them to make a commitment to do so. Participants
were not judged to be more friendly in any one treatment condition, suggesting
that increased thinking and not simply greater liking for the interviewer was
responsible for the results obtained. In addition, the items on which the high
self-disclosure group increased on the nurses' ratings (aware, active, and self-
initiating) seem to reflect a general increased involvement with the environment.

It is significant to note that the memory tests used were measures of short-
term recall, in which there has been some, but by no means unequivocal, evidence
for age-related decline. The study suggests that such decline is not inevitable
and that it can be strongly affected by environmental-social processes. However,
we can only infer that the subjects actually followed the recommended cognitive
activity as a result of the high reciprocal-self-disclosure treatment and that this
led to the memory improvement. Therefore, a second study was designed to
increase, in a very different way, the likelihood that subjects would exercise
their cognitive abilities (Langer et al., 1977).

Whereas the first study provided interpersonal incentives for increased cognitive activity, practical incentives were employed in the second study. Using random assignment to treatment condition, an experimental group for whom positive outcomes depended on remembering was compared with a group for whom positive outcomes were not contingent on memory, and with a no-treatment control group. We predicted that the contingent group would engage in more cognitive activity that would result in improved memory.

We also were interested in learning whether the test context makes a difference in performance. Therefore, for subjects in all three treatment groups, the tests were presented as new kinds of activities that were being tried in the nursing home. Would they find them enjoyable? Would it be more interesting to learn these patterns than watching television? A fourth group was given the same tasks, but they were presented in the standard way, as memory tests. If we combine the performance of the three groups for whom the tasks were presented as a new activity, the pattern recall mean was 4.0 and the probed recall mean was 10.1. In the unconcealed group (for whom we simply said it was a memory test), the pattern recall mean was 2.4 and the probed recall mean was 5.3. Thus it appears that simply describing the nature of the task differently can change performance rather dramatically.

Next let us consider the effects of the manipulation of contingency—the promise of poker chips for remembering information until the next time, with more poker chips leading to a better gift. As Table 10.5 shows, subjects for whom there was a contingency between performance and outcome did significantly better than the subjects for whom there was no contingency for seeking out and remembering this information. On both the probed recall and memory for remote events test, they did significantly better. Clearly there was some generalization of effects, when the intervention was remotivation rather than cognitive instruction.

Other measures showed some further suggestive relationships. The contingent group appeared in slightly better health at two months, although there was no differential effect on vital signs. Interestingly, the complaints went up in the

TABLE 10.5
Summary of All Measures in Study 2

	Memory for meals	Finding out about activities	Lag	Remote events	Health	Vital signs	Complaints
Condition							
Contingent	2.76	12.40	7.50	2.46	5.00	4.31	5.07
Noncontingent	2.20	8.25	4.57	1.53	3.79	4.29	3.64
No treatment			5.83	1.53	3.87	4.21	3.80
p	<.05	<.05	<.01	<.01	<.01	NS	<.001

contingency group. Perhaps if one begins to feel like he or she can do something in the setting, there is an increased action orientation.

While a motivation intervention does appear to enhance cognitive performance, the contingencies have been external in all of the studies that we have considered (prizes and rewards, people who are nice and gain referent power). In such studies, there has been some, but certainly not striking, generalization. Suppose we look, instead, at a memory intervention that made an explicit attempt to teach coping skills and provide incentives that might lead the person to gain internal control. The distinction between learning skills for self-reinforcement and self-regulation, and learning skills to gain external reinforcement may be at the heart of predicting whether we obtain generalization and long-term effects of any of these interventions, be they prevention, alleviation, or enrichment.

In this study (Rodin, 1983), subjects were taught coping skills to improve their performance on a memory task. With instruction from a trained psychologist, they learned how to guide their own performance using cognitive behavioral strategies in a therapy called self-instructional training (Meichenbaum, 1977). Comparing these subjects to subjects who were in an attention control group (they met with the psychologist as often, but they did not get *explicit* training) and to a no-treatment control group, several significant differences emerged in a wide variety of measures. Table 10.6 indicates that in two measures of memory, subjects in the self-instructional group did better than the attention controls. This is essentially a check on the manipulation, since the specific coping

TABLE 10.6
Change Scores From Pre- to Post-Intervention Measures

	Self-instruction	Attention control	No treatment control	F	P
Memory					
Probe recall	19.00	11.66		6.48	<.03
Questions about setting	9.23*	4.88**	4.87**	3.03	<.05
Control					
Control have	51.55**	42.33**	44.87**	3.56	<.03
Value of control (post only)	3.78*	1.44**	1.50**	3.52	<.03
Ideas for change (post only)	3.77*	1.77**	1.12**	5.09	<.01
Activity					
(Percentage of time observed in various activities)					
Passive	20.00*	40.60**	43.90**	2.45	<.09
Active	27.30*	10.60**	10.00**	2.81	<.06
Number of new activities (post only)	1.33**	0.33**	0.67**	2.96	<.05

Note: Numbers with different astericks (*, **, ***) are significantly different from one another.

TABLE 10.7
Change Scores in Pre- to Post-Intervention Measures of Stress Indices

	Self-instruction	Attention control	No treatment control	F	P
Problem stress index					
Pre	1264.6	1343.3	1402.3		
Post	812.4	1238.3	1463.7		
(Change)	(452.2)*	(105.0)*	(−61.4)***	5.62	<.01
Perceived stress index					
Pre	19.4	18.7	19.1		
Post	14.0	15.3	18.7		
(Change)	(5.4)*	(3.4)*	(0.4)**	3.55	<.03

Note: Numbers with different asterisks (*, **, ***) are significantly different from one another.

skills training was with regard to memory skills. But the remainder of the table provides strong evidence for the generalization of these effects. Subjects in the self-instructional group appeared to perceive that they had more control over a variety of aspects of the setting. They had stronger beliefs in the value of trying to exercise control, and they had significantly more ideas for change. There was a slight decline in the number of passive activities and an increase in the number of active activities.

As indicated in Table 10.7, self-instruction subjects appeared to be less stressed on an index measuring the frequency and intensity of problems. Interestingly, all groups receiving attention felt less stressed. Most importantly, as Table 10.8

TABLE 10.8
Change Scores from Pre- to Post Measures on Health Indices

	Self-instruction	Attention control	No treatment control	F	p
Urinary free cortisol (μg/24 hr)					
Pre	112.0	100.8	107.0		
Post (one-month)	62.0	54.5	121.5		
(Change)	(50.0)	(46.3)	(−14.5)	3.38	<.05
Post (18 months)	79.4	93.6	111.5	3.72	<.05
(Change)	(32.6)	(7.2)	(−4.5)		
Physicians' composite ratings					
Pre	26.11	23.88	25.00		
Post (one month)	25.42	26.32	23.96		
(Change)	(.69)	(−2.44)	(1.04)		NS
Post (18 months)	38.33	25.34	24.44		
(Change)	(−12.22)	(−1.46)	(0.56)	4.62	<.02

reveals, there were changes both in urinary free cortisol and in physicians' ratings. While initially there appeared to be nonspecific effects of attention alone, leading to an immediate and substantial decrease in urinary free cortisol in both groups, at the 18-month follow-up there was a much smaller increase in the group given the self-instructional coping skills training as compared to the other two conditions.

The physicians' composite health rating at the immediate one-month post-measure did not show any effect of the intervention, but an analysis of the charts for the 18-month follow-up period showed a clear improvement for the subjects in the coping skills group. These data support the assertion that cognitive interventions that affect subjects' feelings of control may lead to more generalized effects than other types of cognitive interventions.

SOCIAL INTERACTION INTERVENTIONS

There has been a variety of studies, albeit often not very well-controlled, intervening with the families of older persons. This type of intervention is based on the assumption that by bolstering the kind of social support families give, interaction will be less conflicted and more positive, thus leading to better outcomes for older people. These procedures are most widely used when there is a mentally or physically ill older person, but clearly even with the well elderly there are unique family issues that may arise when there is an older family member present. There are few good outcome studies in the enrichment category, and this is an area that is ripe for investigation.

In one study (Hausmen, 1979), support groups for adult children were conducted, aimed at alleviating the transition that they were presumably feeling or going to feel regarding increased responsibility for their older parents. In addition to studying the children, the investigators also studied the parents. They suggested that the elderly parents benefited from an intervention aimed at their children, by showing a decrease in anxiety and depression. The data point to the possibility for improved outcomes by intervening at the family level. Other studies lacking in outcome measures (e.g., Garrison & Howe, 1976) described similar and potentially promising social network interaction interventions, for example where all members of a person's social network, including friends and family, meet together.

The other major type of social intervention strategy involves organized visits to older people. In an interesting study, Laufer and Laufer (1982) developed a program in which local college students received course credit for learning German from a nearby nursing home resident. This intervention took place weekly over the course of a school year. Unfortunately, there were no formal data reported, but descriptions of comments from subjects suggest that their social interaction with other nursing home residents increased and that they experienced an increased feeling of self-worth and purpose as a result of serving in the teacher role. Unfortunately, there were also no control groups, so we can only assume that the mechanism of change was the mutuality of the exchange, rather than being visited per se. Other studies allow us to confirm this inference more strongly.

In a study by Stafford and Bringle (1980), two models of visiting were compared. In one condition, randomly assigned female community residents were visited, and the visit included instruction on completing a kit. From this kit they could make pillows for children who were sick and hospitalized. In a second condition, the visit was entirely social. A third group was a no-treatment control condition. A post-test two weeks after the initial visit revealed that the task group was significantly more interested in increasing their involvement in other activities, such as volunteer work and bingo. These authors suggested that the differences arose because participation in the activity of helping someone else, increased subjects' sense of control and competency, and so increased their incentives to participate in other available activities in the community.

As an experimental test of the importance of control in social interaction, Schulz (1976) organized visits by local college undergraduates to nursing home patients. Subjects were randomly assigned to one of four conditions. One group was given control. This group was allowed to determine the length of the visit and the timing of the visit (i.e., when it would occur). A second group was given predictability—they knew when the next visit would occur, but they did not actually set the time. A third group was given random visits—while they had the same number of visits as subjects in the first two groups, the occurrence of the visits was unpredictable. A fourth group served as a no-treatment control group.

Schulz (1976) measured a variety of psychological and health indicators. As Table 10.9 shows, subjects in both the prediction and the control group were rated as showing greater zest for life compared to the no-treatment and the random-visit groups. They also rated themselves as happier, and, in the control condition, as feeling more useful. On the second measure, the various ratings of health, the strongest difference lay in health status as assessed by the activities director. Again both the prediction and the control groups appeared to improve relative to subjects in the other conditions. These data are shown in Table 10.10. There was also some decrease in the number and types of medications taken from before to after the intervention.

It is important to note that random visits were no better than no visits. The ratings of enjoyment and the ratings of the quality of the random visits suggested that the people did enjoy them (i.e., it was not aversive to have a random visit), but it may be, as Schulz argued, that the generalized benefit of the visits may only come when they are controllable or at least predictable by the individual. At the 24-month follow-up, however, the effects did not maintain themselves. In fact, there was actually a stronger decline for the subjects in the control and predictability groups on almost all measures where they had shown improvement

TABLE 10.9
Mean Psychological Status Indicators by Condition

	Condition			
Variable	No treatment	Random	Predict	Control
"Zest for life" as rated by activities director at home[a]	4.30	5.00	6.10	7.00
Change in level of hope[b]	−.31	−.07	+.20	+.42
Percentage of time lonely	8.00	11.00	3.00	1.00
Percentage of time bored	7.00	15.50	4.00	4.00
Triscale composite on happiness[a]	19.50	20.90	22.70	23.30
Triscale composite on usefulness[d]	17.40	17.50	18.90	21.60

[a]The higher the score, the greater the individual's perceived zest for life.
[b]Positive numbers represent increases, negative numbers decreases.
[c]The higher the score, the more happy the individual perceives himself/herself to be.
[d]The higher the score, the more useful the individual perceives himself/herself to be.

after the intervention. Figures 10.3 and 10.4 show these findings. These are very striking data, especially because mortality also appears to have been affected.

These findings make at least two important points, one practical and one theoretical. At the practical level, it is crucial to plan an intervention that does not withdraw the positive manipulation at the conclusion of the study. Not only were the visits terminated when the study ended, but so were subjects' options for control and predictability. We will return to this point later in the paper. Theoretically, these findings suggest that not all types of control manipulations

TABLE 10.10
Mean Health Status Indicators by Condition

	Condition			
Variable	No treatment	Random	Predict	Control
Health status as assessed by activities director at home[a]	5.10	4.70	6.10	6.90
Triscale composite on health[a]	19.80	20.30	21.20	20.80
Change in number of types of medication taken per day[a]	+.70	+.80	+.40	+.40
Change in quantity of medication taken per day[b]	+2.40	+2.40	+.90	+.80
Change in number of trips to the infirmary per week[b]	+.70	+.85	+.30	+.85

[a]The higher the score, the better the perceived health of the individual.
[b]Positive numbers represent increases.

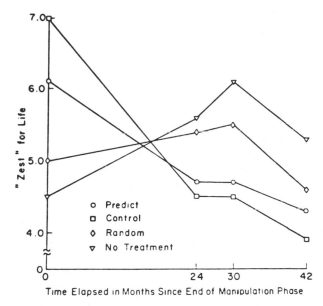

FIGURE 10.3.   Ratings of nursing home patients' zest for life at several time points following control/predictability intervention (from Schulz & Hanusa, 1978).

have the same effects, thus pointing to a need to understand better the construct of control.

MOTIVATION INTERVENTIONS

Our group has viewed control as a motivational variable. Earlier in the chapter we suggested that implicit manipulations of control may have been important in producing generalization of treatment effects; in our studies we developed more explicit manipulations of control in order to influence motivational state.

   In an early study, we (Langer & Rodin, 1976) varied the feelings of control that subjects had over events in a nursing home. The study was intended to determine whether the decline in health, alertness, and activity that generally occurs among the aged in these hospital-like settings could be slowed or reversed by giving them more responsibility for making daily decisions. Subjects in the experimental group had all been randomly assigned to one floor of the nursing home when they entered. They were called together by the hospital administrator and given a talk that said, in part, "We want to tell you the kinds of things that you should be doing, and can be doing, here. There are lots of choices that you can be making; you can decide what you want your rooms to look like, what nights you want to go to the movies, and with whom you want to interact." This

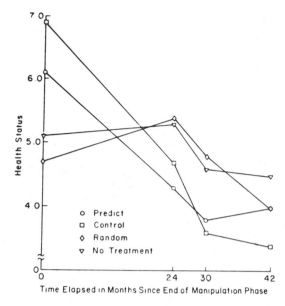

FIGURE 10.4.   Physicians' ratings of nursing home patients' health status at several time points following control/predictability intervention (from Schulz & Hanusa, 1978).

communication emphasized their responsibility for themselves, enumerated things that were possible for them to do in the setting, and explicated where decision making was possible.

A second comparison group was comprised of individuals randomly assigned to another floor of the home. Subjects on the two floors did not differ as a function of severity of illness, prognosis, age, gender, or length of time in the nursing home. These subjects were called together in the same way and were given a talk by the administrator that made explicit what was essentially the implicit message in this nursing home, that it was the staff's responsibility to care for them as patients. They were told, for example, "We want to take care of you, we want you to know that we will do for you whatever you need, so just tell us whenever you need something." While this was a benign, caring communication, it was one that greatly diminished personal control.

In reality, the choices and avenues for decision making that we enumerated in the responsibility condition were options that were already potentially available; the administrator simply stated them clearly as possibilities. Thus, the institutional readiness was there, and the experimental induction was intended to bolster individual predispositions for increased choice and self-control.

The results shown in Table 10.11 indicated that residents in the group given more responsibility became more active and reported feeling less unhappy than the comparison group of residents, which was encouraged to feel that the staff

TABLE 10.11

Mean Scores for Self-Report, Interviewer Ratings, and Nurses' Ratings for
Experimental and Comparison Groups

Questionnaire responses	Responsibility induced (n = 24)			Comparison (n = 28)			Comparison of change scores (p <)
	Pre	Post	Change: Post–Pre	Pre	Post	Change: Post–Pre	
Self-report							
Happy	5.16	5.44	.28	4.90	4.78	−.12	.05
Active	4.07	4.27	.20	3.90	2.62	−1.28	.01
Interviewer rating							
Alertness	5.02	5.31	.29	5.75	5.38	−.37	.025
Nurses' ratings							
General improvement	41.67	45.64	3.97	42.69	40.32	−2.39	.005
Time spent							
Visiting patients	13.03	19.81	6.78	7.94	4.65	−3.30	.005
Visiting others	11.50	13.75	2.14	12.38	8.21	−4.16	.05
Talking to staff	8.21	16.43	8.21	9.11	10.71	1.61	.01
Watching staff	6.78	4.64	−2.14	6.96	11.60	4.64	.05

would care for them and try to satisfy their needs. Patients given responsibility
for making their own decisions also showed significant improvement in alertness
along with increased involvement in many different kinds of activities, such as
attending movies, participating in contests, actively socializing with staff, and
seeking out friends. As indicated in Table 10.12, at an 18-month follow-up,
most of these differences remained.

The health data are shown in Figure 10.5. From a physician's evaluation of
the patients' medical records, it was found that during the 18-month period
following the intervention, the "responsible" patients showed a significantly
greater improvement in health than did the comparable patients in the control
group. The most striking follow-up data were obtained in death-rate differences
between the treatment groups assessed 18 months after the original intervention.
Compared to a 25% mortality rate in that nursing home in the 18 months prior
to the intervention, only 15% in the intervention group died, whereas 30% in
the comparison group died in the 18 months following the study (Rodin & Langer,
1977).

In another motivational manipulation of control, Sherwood and Morris (1980)
randomly assigned subjects to experimental or control groups. Participants were
200 disabled people living in the community. The experimental subjects received
a portable radio transmitter to be worn on their clothing, which when triggered
sent an immediate signal to an emergency response center. This enabled them
to feel control over getting help when they needed it, without relying on family

TABLE 10.12

Mean Ratings for Residents 18 Months Following Experimental
Interventions

Nurses' rating	Responsibility induced (20)[a]	Comparison (14)[a]	No treatment control (9)[b]
Happy	4.35	3.68	3.28
Actively interested	5.15	3.96	3.95
Sociable	5.00	3.78	3.40
Self-initiating	5.15	3.90	4.18
Vigorous	4.75	3.39	3.33

Note: The difference between the responsibility-induced and comparison groups was reliable at $p < .05$ for all ratings but happy. Numbers in parenthesis are *n*s.
[a]Received experimental treatment in Langer and Rodin (1976).
[b]Not previously tested.

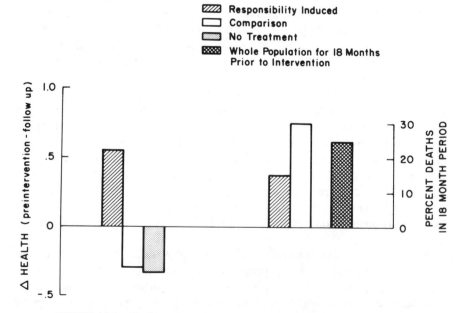

FIGURE 10.5.   Health and mortality at 18-month follow-up for responsibility-induced, comparison, and no-treatment condition subjects.

or friends. As a result of this intervention, experimental subjects exhibited less anxiety, improved sleep patterns, greater confidence in living alone, less use of homemaker services, and delayed entry into nursing homes. The manipulation had no effect on acute hospital or medical services.

Finally, to untangle the inconsistent results of research on relocation, Schulz and Brenner (1977) proposed a model that stressed the importance of control and predictability as mediators of relocation outcomes. Schulz and Hanusa (1977) randomly assigned recently admitted nursing home residents to one of three treatment conditions. To enhance predictability and perceived control, one group received an individualized orientation program that included detailed information about facilities and services available to them, their location within the institution, and directions on how to get to different areas of the hospital. To control for the effects of increased attention, a second group was given the same amount of personal attention but did not receive information designed to make the environment more predictable. A third group served as no-treatment controls. The predictability group was perceived to be healthier than the other two groups following the intervention and to have increased their participation in active activities.

RESOLUTION OF CONFLICTING RESULTS
USING CONTROL INTERVENTIONS

Given the considerable variation in types of control interventions that have been attempted, it will be useful to point out how the differences among them may have produced such different effects—with most studies showing short-term gains and only some showing continued gain after a year or so (e.g., Rodin & Langer, 1977) while others showed greater decline (Schulz & Hanusa, 1978).

Schulz and Hanusa (1978) suggest that Langer and Rodin's (1976) manipulation altered subjects' beliefs about their ability to control outcomes in the setting. The communication delivered to the experimental group, which emphasized their responsibility for themselves and their outcomes, probably encouraged subjects to believe that they themselves could control aspects of the environment. The termination of the experiment had no effect on this view. By contrast, Schulz (1976) manipulated feelings of control over the timing of a visit. In that situation, control was dependent on the presence of an external agent and should not persist once that agent was removed. The Schulz and Hanusa explanation focuses on the importance of subjects perceiving that the locus of control is internal and stable.

A second type of explanation—focusing on environmental and ecological factors—has been advanced by Ransen (1981), who argued that Langer and Rodin's intervention actually changed the setting while Schulz's did not. We suggested in our follow-up paper (Rodin & Langer, 1977) that we set a process in motion by assignment to condition by floor. We did not randomly assign individual subjects to conditions because we were worried about contamination of the manipulation. By conferring treatment on a pre-existing group, we enhanced the probability that not only individuals, but patterns of interaction would be affected systematically. Ransen notes that in our study the agent of change was the director, who was a full time member of that setting, whereas, Schulz used outsiders—the student visitors. Finally our target behaviors had to do with many aspects of the setting, whereas his were limited to the visits. Thus Ransen (1981) argues that interventions in the service of human development are deficient to the extent that they fail to take seriously into account the progressive, mutual accommmodations between people and their physical and social environments.

At first blush this view may present a problem for experiments to test intervention outcomes (i.e., if the direct effects of the intervention cannot be disentangled from any indirect effects attributable to altered patterns of social interaction or any other aspects of the ecology). The problem can be solved, of course, by monitoring the operation of second-order effects instead of trying to eliminate them, especially if one's conceptual model supports the ecological view. These effects may then be analyzed as nested factors within treatment groups (i.e., they may be subjected to statistical as opposed to experimental control). For example, observers could record systematic changes in group interaction, and institutional staff members could be observed periodically to assess changes in their practices and attitudes. Such studies have not yet been attempted.

CONCLUSION

After reviewing the studies described above, we conclude that it is possible to do well-controlled field experiments but that relatively few exist at present. Nonetheless, data thus far suggest the practical contribution of such studies, especially those based on theoretical models. Enrichment studies in particular support the life span developmental view and reinforce suggestions that there is both great variability and great plasticity in the aging process. Individual control and salutary environmental experiences appear to be important mediators in this developmental process. Indeed, we may conclude from most of the studies we have reviewed that for the maintenance of the positive effects of enrichment interventions, one or both of the following is/are necessary: They must (1) influence the subjects' own self-regulatory skills and perceived control, and/or (2) change the context to promote more adaptive behavior. Most intriguingly, some of these studies are beginning to suggest that psychosocial interventions may impact on biological as well as psychological outcomes.

ACKNOWLEDGMENT

Preparation of the paper was supported by NIA Grant AG02455.

REFERENCES

Baltes, P. B. (1973, Spring). Strategies for psychological intervention in old age: A symposium. *Gerontologist, 13*(1), 4–6.

Brickman, P., Rabinowitz, V. C., Karuza, J., Coates, D., Cohn, E., & Kidder, L. (1982). Models of helping and coping. *American Psychologist, 37*, 368–384.

Canestrari, R. E. (1968). Age changes in acquisition. In G. A. Taland (Ed.), *Human aging and behavior*. New York: Academic Press. New York, 1968.

Craik, F. I. M. (1977). Age differences in human memory. In J. E. Birren & K. W. Schaie (Eds.), *Handbook of the psychology of aging*. New York: Van Nostrand Reinhold.

Fozard, J. L., & Popkin, S. J. (1978). Optimizing adult development: Ends and means of an applied psychology of aging. *American Psychologist*, 975–989.

Frank, J. D. (1976). Restoration of morale and behavioral change. In A. Burton (Ed.), *What makes behavior change possible?* New York: Brunner/Mazel.

French, J. R. P., Jr., & Raven, B. H. (1959). The bases of social power. In D. Cartwright (Ed.), *Studies in social power*. Ann Arbor: University of Michigan.

Garrison, J. E., & Howe, J. (1976). Community intervention with the elderly: A social network approach. *Journal of the American Geriatrics Society, 24*, 329–333.

Gatz, M., Popkin, S. J., Pino, C. D., VandenBos, G. R. (1985). Psychological interventions with older adults. In J. E. Birren & K. W. Schaie (Eds.), *Handbook of the psychology of aging* (2nd ed., pp. 755–785). New York: Van Nostrand Reinhold.

Gurland, B. J., Fleiss, J. L., Goldberg, K., Sharpe, L., Copeland, J. R. M., Kelleher, M. J., & Kellet, J. M. (1976). The geriatric mental state schedule. II. Factor analysis. *Psychological Medical, 6*, 451–459.

Hausmen, C. P. (1979). Short-term counseling groups for people with elderly parents. *The Gerontologist, 19*, 102–107.

Horn, J. L. (1972). State, trait and change dimensions of intelligence. *British Journal of Educational Psychology, 42*, 159–185.

Horn, J. L. (1978). Organization of data on life-span development of human abilities. In L. R. Goulet & P. B. Baltes (Eds.), *Life-span developmental psychology: Research and theory*. New York: Academic Press, 1978.

Horn, J. L., & Cattell, R. B. (1967). Age differences in fluid and crystallized intelligence. *Acta Psychologica, 26*, 107–129.

Hughston, G. A., & Merriam, S. B. (1982). Reminiscence: A nonformal technique for improving cognitive functioning in the aged. *International Journal of Aging and Human Development, 15*, 139–149.

Hulicka, J. M., & Grossman, J. L. (1967). Age-group comparisons for the use of mediators in paired-associates learning. *Journal of Gerontology, 22*, 46–51.

Hultsch, D. (1969). Adult age differences in the organization of free recall. *Developmental Psychology, 1*, 673–678.

Hultsch, D. (1975). Adult age difference in retrieval: Trace development and dependant forgetting. *Developmental Psychology, 11*, 197–201.

Jacobs, A. (1972). Strategies of social intervention: Past and future. In A. Jacobs & W. Spradlin (Eds.), *The group as agent of change*. Chicago: Aldine.

Janis, I. L., & Rodin, J. (1979). Attributions, control and decision making: Social psychology and health care. In G. Stone, F. Cohen, & N. Adler (Eds.), *Health psychology*, San Francisco: Jossey-Bass.

Kahn, R. L., & Antonucci, T. C. (1981). Convoys of social support: A life course approach. In S. B. Kiesler, J. N. Morgan & V. K. Oppenheimer (Eds.), *Aging: Social change*. New York: Academic Press.

Kahn, R. L., Zarit, S. H., Hilbert, N. M., & Niederehe, G. (1975). Memory complaint and impairment in the aged: The effects of depression and altered brain function. *Archives of General Psychiatry, 32*, 1569–1573.

Langer, E., & Rodin, J. (1976). The effects of choice and enhanced personal responsibility: A field experiment in an institutional setting. *Journal of Personality and Social Psychology, 34*, 191–198.

Langer, E. J., Rodin, J., Beck, P., & Weinman, C., & Spitzer, L. (1979). Environmental determinants of memory improvement in late adulthood. *Journal of Personality and Social Psychology, 37*, 2003–2013.

Laufer, E. A., & Laufer, W. S. (1982). From geriatric resident to language professor: A new program using the talents of the elderly in a skilled nursing facility. *The Gerontologist, 22*, 548–550.

Lowenthal, M. F., Thurner, M., & Chiriboga, D. (1975). *Four stages of life. A psychological study of men and women facing transitions*. San Francisco: Jossey–Bass.

Meichenbaum, D. (1977). *Cognitive-behavior modification*. New York: Plenum Press.

Perlmutter, M. (1978). What is memory aging the aging of? *Developmental Psychology, 14*, 330–345.

Perrotta, P., & Meacham, J. A. (1981–1982). Can a reminiscing intervention alter depression and self-esteem? *International Journal of Aging and Human Development, 14*, 23–30.

Plemons, J. K., Willis, S. L., & Baltes, P. P. (1978). Modifiability of fluid intelligence in aging: A short-term longitudinal training approach. *Journal of Gerontology, 33*, 224–231.

Poon, L. W., Fozard, J. L., & Treat, N. J. (1978). From clinical and research findings on memory to intervention programs. *Experimental Aging Research, 4*, 235–253.

Ransen, D. L. (1981). Long-term effects of two interventions with the aged: An ecological analysis. *Journal of Applied Developmental Psychology, 2*, 13–27.

Rodin, J. (1983). Behavioral medicine: Beneficial effects of self control training in aging. *International Review of Applied Psychology, 32*, 153–181.

Rodin, J., & Langer, E. (1977). Long-term effect of a control-relevant intervention. *Journal of Personality and Social Psychology, 35*, 897.

Schulz, R. (1976). Effects of control and predictability on the physical and psychological well-being of the institutionalized aged. *Journal of Personality and Social Psychology, 33*, 563–573.

Schulz, R., & Brenner, G. F. (1977). Relocation of the aged: A review and theoretical analysis. *Journal of Gerontology, 32*, 323–333.

Schulz, R., & Hanusa, B. H. (1977, November). *Facilitating institutional adaptation of the aged: Effects of predictability-enhancing intervention*. Paper presented at the meeting of the American Gerontological Society, San Francisco.

Schulz, R., & Hanusa, B. H. (1978). Long-term effects of control and predictability-enhancing interventions: Findings and ethical issues. *Journal of Personality and Social Psychology, 36*, 1194–1201.

Sherwood, S., & Morris, L. (1980). Lifeline signalling devices and health outcomes. Unpublished report, Boston University.

Stafford, J. L., & Bringle, R. (1980). The influence of task success on elderly women's interest in new activities. *The Gerontologist, 20*, 642–648.

Taylor, S. E., & Fiske, S. T. (1978). Salience, attention, and attribution: Top of the head phenomena. In L. Berkowitz (Ed.), *Advances in experimental social psychology*. New York: Academic Press.

Treat, N. J., & Reese, H. W. (1976). Age, pacing, and imagery in paired-associate learning. *Developmental Psychology, 12*, 119–124.

Zarit, S. H., Cole, K. D., & Guider, R. L. (1981). Memory training strategies and subjective complaints of memory in the aged. *The Gerontologist, 21*, 158–164.

AUTHOR INDEX

SUBJECT INDEX